Lipids and Heart Disease

A Guide for the Primary Care Team

SECOND EDITION

MADELEINE BALL

*Professor, School of Nutrition and
Public Health, Deakin University,
Melbourne, Australia*

and

JIM MANN

*Professor, Departments of Human Nutrition and Medicine,
University of Otago, New Zealand*

Oxford   Auckland   New York   Tokyo
OXFORD UNIVERSITY PRESS
1994

Oxford University Press, Walton Street, Oxford OX2 6DP

Oxford   New York
Athens   Auckland   Bangkok   Bombay
Calcutta   Cape Town   Dar es Salaam   Delhi
Florence   Hong Kong   Istanbul   Karachi
Kuala Lumpur   Madras   Madrid   Melbourne
Mexico City   Nairobi   Paris   Singapore
Taipei   Tokyo   Toronto
and associated companies in
Berlin   Ibadan

Oxford is a trade mark of Oxford University Press

Published in the United States
by Oxford University Press Inc., New York

A catalogue record for this book is available from the British Library

Library of Congress Cataloging in Publication Data
Ball, Madeleine.
Lipids and heart disease: a guide for the primary care team/
Madeleine Ball and Jim Mann.—2nd ed.
(Oxford medical publications)
Includes bibliographical references.
1. Hyperlipidemia.   2. Coronary heart disease—Etiology.
I. Mann, Jim.   II. Title.   III. Series.
[DNLM: 1. Coronary Disease— etiology.   2. Lipids—adverse effects.
3. Coronary Disease—prevention & control.   4. Hyperlipidemia—
diagnosis.   5. Hyperlipidemia—prevention & control.   WG 300 B187L 1994]
RC632.H87B35   1994   616.1'23071–dc20   94–3341
ISBN 0 19 262495 4

Typeset by EXPO Holdings, Malaysia.

Printed in Great Britain by
Redwood Books, Trowbridge, Wilts

Introduction

Coronary heart disease (CHD) is a major cause of death in most countries of the Western world. In 1990, almost 160 000 people in the UK died of CHD. Over 30 per cent of all male deaths are from CHD. Each year about 30 000 of the men who die are under age 65 and 5000 are under age 55. Fig. 1 shows the overall causes of death in men and women.

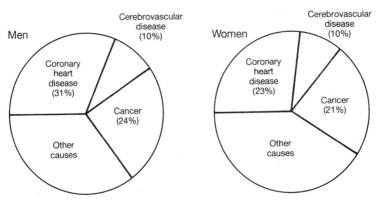

Fig. 1 Overall cause of death in the UK as a percentage of the total.

The British Regional Heart Study showed that by age 55–59 almost one in three men had symptoms or signs of CHD. Death rates from CHD vary between different countries, as shown in Table 1. In New Zealand in 1988, 26 per cent of all deaths were attributable to CHD, and the various causes of death in men and women aged 45–64 are shown in Fig. 2.

The death rate from CHD at age 30–69 has been falling in a number of countries, particularly the USA, Australia and New Zealand, and to a lesser extent in England and Wales. The rates are, however, rising in many eastern European countries, as shown in Fig. 3.

The major risk factors for CHD include smoking, hypertension, and raised blood lipids. Surveys in many countries, including Britain,

Table 1.   Age standard mortality from CHD—ages 35–74 (1988)

	Deaths per 100 000 men
Northern Ireland	658
USSR	596
Finland	557
England and Wales	490
Australia	374
USA	339
France	137
Japan	62

Australia, and New Zealand, have shown that these risk factors are common. Much has been written in the last 15 years about the importance of lipids, particularly cholesterol, in determining CHD risk. The variation in CHD between populations is largely explained by differences in cholesterol levels. The large number of people with a plasma cholesterol concentration above 'ideal' can thus contribute towards the high incidence of CHD. In populations with a high CHD risk, increased plasma cholesterol contributes to CHD incidence in two

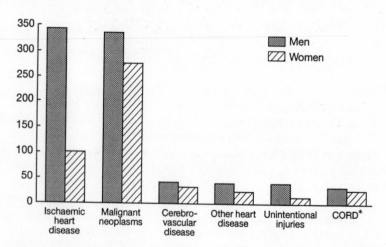

Fig. 2   Selected major causes of death in people aged 45–64, 1988—rates per 100 000 population. *Chronic obstructive respiratory disease.

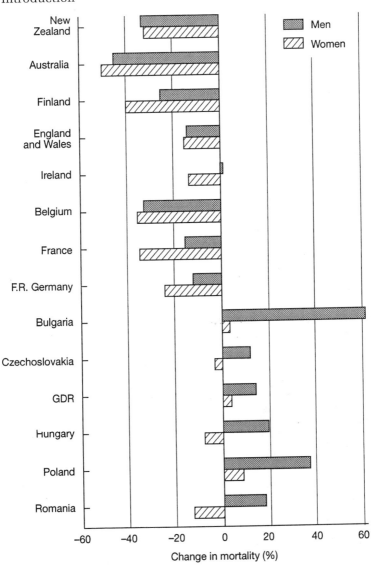

Fig. 3 Changes in CHD mortality (per cent)—1970–85 age-standardized figures for men and women aged 30–69.

ways. First, there are a large number of people (probably half the population) with a slight to moderate increase in plasma lipid levels which result in some increase in risk of CHD. Second, there is a smaller group of people with high levels, often due to an inherited disorder, who are at particularly high risk for premature CHD (Fig. 3).

Plasma concentrations of cholesterol and triglyceride which are higher than ideal result from a number of causes. Some are primary, due to a specific disorder of lipid metabolism, and others are secondary, where abnormalities in lipid metabolism result from another condition. The 'Western lifestyle', associated with obesity and a diet high in saturated fat, appears to be the main cause of the large number of people with a high cholesterol level in a population. However, genetic influences also play a part. Conditions such as familial hypercholesterolaemia, which is due to a single gene defect, cause markedly raised plasma cholesterol levels and a very high CHD risk. At least one in 500 people in Britain has this condition, and there are other inherited conditions which are even commoner. Polygenic factors also appear important and probably explain why some people have higher lipid levels than others despite eating a similar diet.

Epidemiological studies have shown that the risk of cardiovascular disease steadily increases with increasing levels of plasma cholesterol and that it is difficult to define a 'healthy' range. Many people at the upper end of the statistically defined 'normal' range are at far greater risk than those with lower levels and it is for this reason that the World Health Organization and many national organizations have recommended dietary change for the entire population. The epidemiological evidence for the value of population dietary change is strong. There are also clinical trials which show that both cardiovascular morbidity and mortality are reduced as a result of treating hyperlipidaemia, and that the identification and treatment of individuals with an inherited hyperlipidaemia is likely to be particularly beneficial.

This book discusses the contribution of lipids and other risk factors to the current epidemic of CHD. It covers the causes of CHD and its epidemiology, the investigation and management of hyperlipidaemia, and the means by which CHD may be reduced in the population. For convenience it is divided into sections which can be read independently.

Melbourne   M. B.
Dunedin   J. M.
July 1994

Acknowledgements

We thank the general practitioners who initially encouraged us to write this book. Dr I. Robertson contributed Chapter 12.

Contents

Glossary

Apolipoproteins (apoproteins)—protein components of lipoproteins that are involved in structure, cell recognition, and the metabolism of the lipoproteins.

Lipoproteins—lipids are insoluble in water, and are therefore transported in plasma in particles containing various proportions of protein, phospholipid, triglyceride, and cholesterol.

VLDL—very low density lipoprotein
IDL —intermediate density lipoprotein
LDL —low density lipoprotein
HDL —high density lipoprotein

classification based on centrifugation data

Non-esterified fatty acid—single fatty acid molecules. Three of these in combination with glycerol form a triglyceride molecule.

Saturated fatty acids—these are fatty acids with no double bonds in the carbon skeleton. Stearic and palmitic acids are the commonest; high levels of these are found in most hard animal fats.

Monounsaturated fatty acids—fatty acids with a single unsaturated $C = C$ bond e.g. oleic acid. Olive oil is rich in this fatty acid.

Polyunsaturated fatty acids—fatty acids with multiple $C = C$ bonds e.g. linoleic acid. Sunflower seed, soya, and corn oil contain considerable quantities of these fatty acids.

Units—cholesterol 1 mmol/l $\simeq$ 39 mg/dl; triglyceride 1 mmol/l $\simeq$ 88 mg/dl

Section I

Coronary heart disease: the role of lipids

1

The function of lipids

Although raised levels of lipids in the circulation are associated with coronary heart disease, triglycerides, phospholipids, and cholesterol have extremely important functions in the body.

Triglycerides

Triglycerides of both plant and animal origin are a major dietary energy source. They comprise 95 per cent of the lipids in adipose tissue and are a source of energy during periods of starvation (Table 1.1).

During periods of adequate feeding, triglycerides can be synthesized in the body and stored.

Table 1.1   Energy stores in adults

	Storage form	Energy provision (resting state)
Carbohydrate	Glycogen in liver and muscle	6–12 hours
Amino acids	Protein, mainly in skeletal muscle	10–18 days
Triglyceride	Fat in adipose tissue	20–30 days

Phospholipids

These are the fundamental components of cell membranes.

Cholesterol

This is an important component of plasma membranes and lipoproteins, primarily regulating their fluidity and stability. It is a precursor of bile

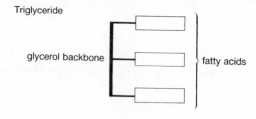

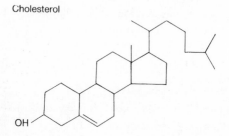

Fig. 1.1 Diagrammatic representation of a triglyceride and a cholesterol molecule.

acids and steroid hormones. Dietary cholesterol comes largely from eggs and dairy produce, and diets with a high saturated fat content are generally high in cholesterol. The average intake in people eating Western diets is 300 to 500 mg per day, but some people have as much as 1000 mg. Cholesterol is also synthesized in the body and is excreted in bile salts and bile as free cholesterol. Figure 1.1 shows both a triglyceride and a cholesterol molecule.

Lipoproteins

Triglycerides and other lipids are insoluble in plasma and circulate as particles called lipoproteins which contain triglyceride, cholesterol, phospholipid, and proteins. These proteins, called apolipoproteins, help to regulate the structure and interactions of the lipoproteins. Fat metabolism is described in the Appendix, but an outline is given below and Fig. 1.2 is simplified diagram of lipoprotein metabolism.

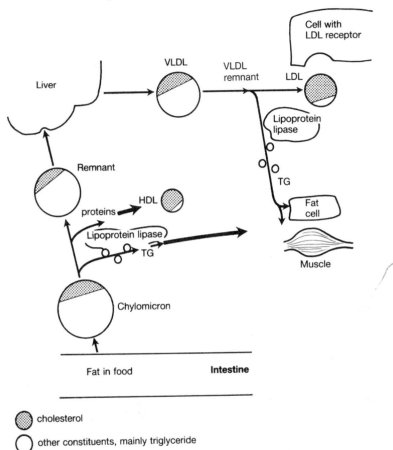

Fig. 1.2 Simplified outline of lipoprotein metabolism.

Fat absorption

Fats constitute 40 per cent of the energy intake of many people. Partial hydrolysis of fats occurs in the small intestine; monoglycerides and fatty acids are absorbed and then re-esterified in the mucosal cells to form triglycerides. Cholesterol is also absorbed in the small intestine and combines with triglycerides, phospholipids, and specific apolipoproteins in the intestinal cells. The chylomicrons formed are rich in triglyceride and are secreted into the lymphatic system.

Chylomicrons and very low density lipoprotein

Chylomicrons enter the blood stream via the lymphatic system and may cause the plasma to become turbid.

Another triglyceride-rich lipoprotein, VLDL, is synthesized in the liver, and its triglyceride component is derived from circulating fatty acids and excess dietary carbohydrate.

In the circulation, triglyceride is gradually removed from both chylomicrons and VLDL by the action of lipoprotein lipase, which is present in the capillaries of a number of tissues, but predominantly in adipose tissue and skeletal muscle. The glycerides and fatty acids removed are taken up by muscle or adipose cells. They provide the main energy source for aerobic metabolism in muscle, and in a well-fed individual the excess is stored as triglyceride. As triglycerides are removed the remnant particle becomes smaller and some surface components transfer to HDL particles. The chylomicron remnant is then generally taken up by the liver and the VLDL remnant becomes LDL.

Low density lipoprotein

LDL is a cholesterol-rich particle. In healthy people over half the LDL enters the cells after binding with high-affinity cell receptors and, once in the cell, is degraded to liberate the cholesterol. There is also a receptor independent pathway, which becomes proportionally more important at higher LDL concentrations. The activity of the high-affinity receptor is a major determinant of plasma LDL and cholesterol levels, and disorders affecting these receptors, such as familial hypercholesterolaemia, result in greatly increased levels.

High density lipoproteins

The other group of lipoproteins in the circulation are the heterogeneous HDL particles (HDL_1, HDL_2, and HDL_3). These contain cholesterol and several apolipoproteins with various functions, some poorly understood. They represent a pool of re-usable apolipoproteins, and appear to be involved in the retrograde transport of cholesterol from peripheral tissues to the liver.

Lipoprotein (a)

$Lp_{(a)}$ is an altered form of LDL with a large glycoprotein, $apo_{(a)}$, disulphide bonded to the apo B_{100} moiety of LDL. The protein bears a strong resemblance to plasminogen, and may be atherogenic by interfering with plasminogen or LDL metabolism. $Lp_{(a)}$ levels are a risk factor for coronary heart disease and stroke.

Hyperlipidaemia

A high concentration of circulating lipoproteins usually results from an increase in their synthesis due to a diet high in saturated fat, and/or a genetically determined reduction in the removal from the circulation. Depending on the type of particles this causes an increase in the concentration of cholesterol and/or triglyceride in the plasma.

2

Plasma lipids and coronary heart disease

What are normal lipid levels?

Many departments of chemical pathology provide a normal or reference range in brackets after the result of a requested biochemical measurement. We have become accustomed to passing any results which lie within this range as satisfactory. However, it is not always appreciated that the normal range is a statistical concept based upon two standard deviations above and below the mean level of a group of apparently healthy people from the population. For most biochemical measurements the statistical normal range is equivalent to an optimal range, but this does not apply to measurements of blood lipids. What is an acceptable range, instead of the 'normal' range, is the reference against which a person's results need to be considered, and an indication of this is now provided by many laboratories.

Total plasma cholesterol: relationship to coronary heart disease (CHD)

No other blood constituent varies so much between different populations as the plasma cholesterol. From New Guinea to East Finland, the mean plasma cholesterol ranges from 2.6 to 7.1 mmol/l (100–275 mg/dl) when estimated by the same method in the same age and sex group.

Relationship between populations

The extent to which total cholesterol explains the geographic variation of CHD varies in different studies. The effect appeared to be particularly strong in the Seven Countries Study carried out by Keys and coworkers. These researchers measured actual food consumption and various factors known to be related to CHD (including cigarette smoking, blood pressure, obesity, and plasma cholesterol) in 16 groups of people living in seven countries and followed each group to determine 10-year incidence rates of CHD. As shown in Fig. 2.1, median cholesterol values were highly correlated with CHD death rates (r = 0.80) and cholesterol accounted for 64 per cent of the variance in the CHD death rates among the groups. Dietary saturated fat intake was

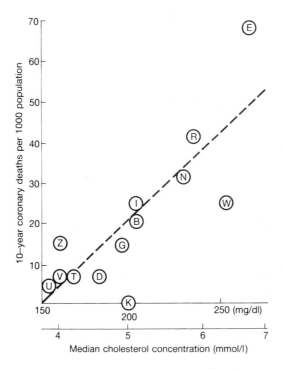

Fig. 2.1 Relationship between the mean cholesterol in different countries and CHD death rates. The relationship of the median plasma cholesterol level to 10-year CHD mortality in 16 male cohorts of the Seven Countries Study. B = Belgrade (Yugoslavia); D = Dalmatia (Yugoslavia); E = East Finland; G = Corfu; I = Italian railroad; K = Crete; N = Zutphen (Holland); T = Tanushimaru (Japan); R = American railroad; U = Ushibuka (Japan); V = Velike Krsna (Yugoslavia); W = West Finland; Z = Zrenjanin (Yugoslavia). (From Keys, A. (1980). *Seven countries. A multivariate analysis of death and coronary heart disease*. Harvard University Press.)

also strongly correlated with cholesterol and with 10-year CHD mortality. Interestingly, none of the other factors known to be related to CHD (cigarette smoking, blood pressure, obesity, and physical inactivity) explained the geographical variation of CHD to any appreciable extent. This suggests that the emergence of CHD in a community depends strongly upon the cholesterol level of the community and that the other factors become important only when the population is at risk because of increased cholesterol levels. On the other hand, in the MONICA/WHO study which included a greater number of countries, the classical risk factors (cholesterol, blood pressure, and smoking) accounted for a smaller proportion of the variation in CHD rates and other factors such as the levels of antioxidants eg. vitamin E in the blood also played an important role in determining the geographic variation in CHD. However, of marked importance is the fact that among individuals within populations the association between CHD and plasma cholesterol is strong.

Within populations

In over 20 prospective studies in different countries total serum cholesterol has been shown to be related to the development of CHD. The association occurs in both sexes and is independent of all other measured risk factors. The relationship in the largest prospective study of over 350 000 people is shown in Fig. 2.2. A clear 'dose-related' effect is apparent with a gradient of risk from the lowest to the highest levels. There is no discernable critical value below which there is no risk; the risk tends to increase throughout the range. Multiple measurements of serum cholesterol in an individual improve the accuracy of assessment of cholesterol-mediated risk and predict an appreciably greater degree of risk than single measurements.

Comparison of groups of people within one population who eat different diets, shows that diet has some effect, although it does not fully explain the lipid levels within populations. Figure 2.3 shows that vegans, vegetarians, and those who eat fish but no meat, have lower levels of cholesterol than meat eaters within the British population. These groups have been found to have lower rates of CHD than meat eaters and this may be explained at least in part by the lower cholesterol levels. Diet thus appears to exert a profound effect, influencing both the differences in cholesterol levels and CHD rates among populations and among groups with different dietary practices living within high-risk populations.

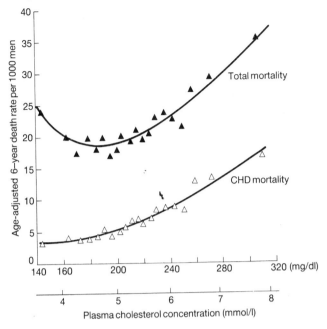

Fig. 2.2 Relationship between plasma cholesterol and CHD-MRFIT Study. (Martin, M. *et al.* (1986). *Lancet*, **2**, 933–6.)

Reference range versus optimal levels

The distribution of cholesterol levels has been examined in a number of different countries. The 'normal' or reference range (based on two standard deviations above and below the mean), calculated from the cholesterol levels of 25–59-year-olds in the British National Lipid Screening Project, is from 3.5–8.0 mmol/l (Fig. 2.4). Similar ranges are found in most other affluent societies. It is thus clear that for cholesterol 'normal' certainly does not imply 'optimal'. Those at the upper end of the range have a greater risk of CHD than those at the bottom. Under these circumstances it is clearly desirable to try to define an optimal range. As with other biological variables showing a gradient of risk (such as blood pressure) this is not an easy task.

Various national and international organizations have suggested that a cholesterol level of 5.2 mmol/l or less should be regarded as a desirable level for individual adults within high-risk populations and a target

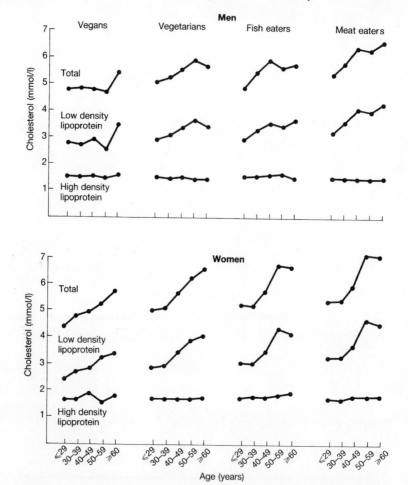

Fig. 2.3 Plasma cholesterol concentration and dietary habits. (Thorogood *et al.* (1987). *British Medical Journal*, **295**, 351–4.)

population level in such countries where average levels are almost invariably appreciably greater than this. Concentrations of 6.5 and 7.5 mmol/l have often been regarded as levels above which individuals should respectively receive individual advice or be considered for drug therapy. The proportion of the British population with cholesterol levels greater than these cut-off points is shown in Fig. 2.5 and statis-

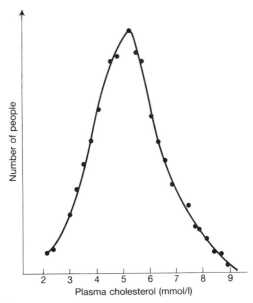

Fig. 2.4 Distribution of plasma cholesterol concentrations found in the British National Lipid Screening Project. (Mann, J. *et al.* (1988). *British Medical Journal*, **296**, 1702–6.)

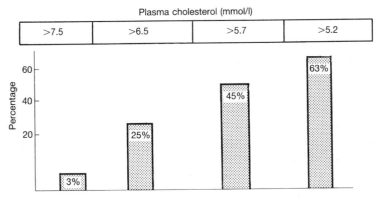

Fig. 2.5 Plasma cholesterol levels in the British population, 1987.

tics in other countries are comparable. However there is growing realization that degree of risk conferred by a particular level of cholesterol is determined by the presence of other risk factors and whether or not the individual has already developed CHD. This issue needs to be taken into account when considering guidelines for the management of hyperlipidaemia and is discussed further in Chapter 11.

Overall cholesterol levels are not appreciably different in men and women, but different age trends are apparent. In the younger age groups, women have lower levels than men. However, there is a steady gradient for both total and LDL cholesterol with increasing age in women, as shown in Fig. 2.6, which may partly explain the rapid rise in CHD after the menopause. Levels in men generally increase only until the mid-forties after which they tend to level off. It is this observation that has led some people to suggest that the advisable and 'action limits' for plasma cholesterol should be age- and sex-adjusted. We do not know if this is sensible because it is not yet clear whether a raised cholesterol confers a different risk at different ages. The increase with age is less marked in populations with lower mean cholesterol levels.

The effect of particularly low plasma cholesterol

The inverse relationship between cholesterol and total non-cardiovascular mortality at the lower end of the range (Fig. 2.2) was initially used as an argument against the suggestion that the lowest cholesterol levels were the most satisfactory. There appears to be an increased risk of non-cardiovascular deaths (chiefly from cancer) in those with the lowest plasma cholesterol. Most studies show that this inverse association is confined to deaths in the very early years of follow-up and it is now generally believed that the low cholesterol in some of these individuals was a metabolic consequence of the cancer which was present, but unsuspected, at the time of the initial examination. Further evidence against an unfavourable effect of low plasma cholesterol comes from cross-cultural comparisons: countries with a low population mean cholesterol not only have low CHD rates, but also show no evidence of any increased risk of cancer.

Low density lipoprotein cholesterol

The association of total cholesterol with CHD morbidity and mortality appears to derive chiefly, if not entirely, from the LDL cholesterol frac-

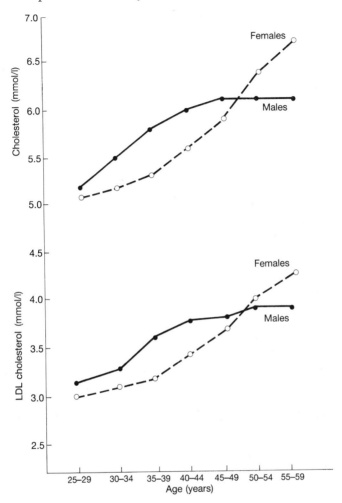

Fig. 2.6 Relationship between total and LDL cholesterol, sex, and age.

tion with which it is very highly correlated. Unfortunately, LDL cholesterol has been measured in relatively few epidemiological studies and
there are no clearly defined, internationally accepted, optimal ranges.
What is apparent though is that levels greater than 5.0 mmol/l, in
adults, are associated with a considerable CHD risk, and that most individuals with familial hypercholesterolaemia have levels above this.

The mean LDL cholesterol levels, at different ages, seen in the British National Lipid Screening Project are shown in Fig. 2.6. In this study the LDL cholesterol was calculated from the measurements of total cholesterol, HDL cholesterol, and triglycerides using the Friedewald equation (see Chapter 5).

Recent case control studies have suggested that LDL particle size may be a particularly important determinant of premature CHD risk. Small, dense, low molecular weight LDL particles were more prevalent in men with premature CHD than controls, to the extent that these small particles have been associated with a three-fold increase in risk of myocardial infarction. These small LDL particles are also more susceptible to oxidation which enhances their atherogenic potential (see Chapter 3).

High density lipoprotein cholesterol

HDL has been repeatedly shown to be a protective factor against CHD in both case–control and prospective studies. Women have higher HDL levels than men and a lower CHD risk. HDL levels remain relatively constant with age. Low HDL may be particularly predictive of CHD risk in women. It is the HDL_2 subfraction that appears to be most important in terms of 'protection'. Some studies have shown the predictive value of low HDL to be stronger than that associated with high LDL in people over 50 years. Low HDL may be associated with obesity, cigarette smoking, lack of physical activity, impaired glucose tolerance (IGT), or NIDDM as well as genetic predisposition and some prospective studies suggested that the protective effect is not independent when controlling for the effects of other risk factors. However a recent analysis of four large American prospective studies suggests that an increment of 1 mg/100 ml (0.026 mmol/) is associated with a 2–3 per cent reduction in CHD. When attempting to build up a detailed lipid risk profile it is appropriate to measure both LDL and HDL.

Plasma triglycerides and VLDL

The study of plasma triglycerides is complicated by the fact that levels show a marked variation in response to meals. It is usual to study fasting levels and the fasting plasma triglyceride related to age and sex is shown in Fig. 2.7. The reference interval calculated from these data is 0.5–1.8 mmol/l. Markedly raised plasma triglyceride concentrations,

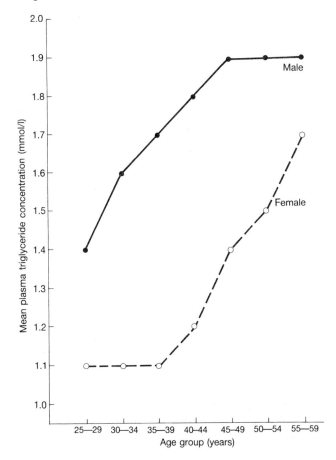

Fig. 2.7 Fasting plasma triglyceride concentrations. (Data from British National Lipid Screening Project.)

to above 15–20 mmol/l, are associated with a risk of acute pancreatitis. High triglyceride levels may also be associated with an increased thrombotic tendency in any artery, and this may occur even in the absence of marked atherosclerosis.

The situation with regard to more modest elevations of triglyceride is more complex. Increases in total triglycerides and levels of VLDL

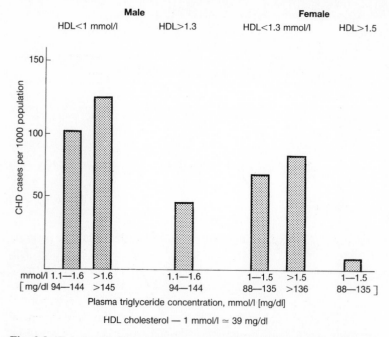

Fig. 2.8 Relationship between plasma triglyceride concentration, HDL, and CHD.

triglycerides are usually associated with increased CHD rates in prospective studies, though without the clear graded increase in risk seen for cholesterol. The extent to which the increased risk is independent of other measures of lipid metabolism has not been clearly established. A relatively recent analysis of the Framingham data (Table 2.1) suggests that raised levels of triglyceride are associated with CHD risk only in the presence of reduced levels of HDL (Fig. 2.8). Case–control studies suggest that 'abnormal' VLDL (i.e. relative cholesterol enriched VLDL) may be a particularly important predictor of premature CHD. Thus measurement of total triglyceride and VLDL undertaken in most of the prospective studies may be insufficiently sensitive to determine the extent to which this component of the lipoprotein mediated risk predicts CHD. Further studies which include measurement of VLDL composition may be required.

Table 2.1   Levels of high density lipoprotein (HDL) cholesterol and subsequent incidence of ischaemic heart disease in the Framingham study

HDL cholesterol (mmol/l)	CHD rate/1000 population
All levels	77
<0.65	177
0.65–1.38	103
1.40–1.64	54
1.64–1.90	25

Summary

Unlike other biochemical measurements that are frequently performed, lipid levels within the 'normal' range are not necessarily optimal. For cholesterol and LDL the 'ideal' range is much lower than the 'normal' range. There appears to be little risk associated with plasma triglyceride levels which are a little over the upper end of the reference range, but the effect seems to depend on the HDL level. Some of the more important 'normal' ranges and the suggested optimal range are summarized in Table 2.2. Most affluent societies have cholesterol and LDL levels which are appreciably greater than optimal and HDL levels which are lower. It seems likely that if optimal levels could be achieved then the risk of CHD would be appreciably reduced. Evidence for the benefit of cholesterol lowering comes from epidemiological studies as well as from the clinical trials discussed in Chapter 4. In the future, measurements of LDL particle size and VLDL composition may improve the prediction of lipoprotein mediated risk of CHD.

Table 2.2   Reference and suggested 'healthy' ranges for plasma cholesterol, LDL, and HDL cholesterol (mmol/l) and triglycerides (mmol/l) for adults under 60 years

	Reference	Suggested
Total cholesterol	3.5–7.8	<5.5
LDL cholesterol	2.3–6.1	<4.0
HDL cholesterol	0.8–1.7	>1.15
Triglycerides	0.7–1.8	0.7–1.7

Note   The reference interval is the interval calculated from the mean of an apparently healthy population plus and minus two standard deviations.

3

Atherosclerosis: the process and the risk factors

The basic pathology underlying the development of CHD, and other vascular disease, in patients with hyperlipidaemia is nearly always atherosclerosis. Atherosclerosis tends to affect large- and medium-sized arteries such as the aorta and the femoral, coronary, and cerebral arteries, and is common at sites of turbulent blood flow such as arterial bifurcations. As atherosclerosis develops over many years it is not possible to follow the process closely, and there has been great debate as to its pathogenesis.

A current concept of the pathogenesis of atherosclerosis is called the modified response to injury hypothesis. The process is considered to be proliferative, rather than primarily degenerative, and is believed to begin early in life. An accumulation of monocytes and lipid-filled macrophages can be found in the coronary arteries before the age of 10 and this increases during adolescence. The juvenile fatty streak consists of lipid-filled monocytes and macrophages within the intima of the vessel. It occurs, however, in children in all societies, including those in which adult atherosclerosis is rare, and it is controversial whether these lesions progress to fibrous plaques.

Fibrous plaques are white lesions which often protrude into the vessel lumen. The lipid, which is mainly derived from plasma lipoproteins, forms a core, along with necrotic cells, and is covered by a fibrous layer. In advanced lesions, calcium is deposited and thrombus is often present. At least four cell types participate in the formation of an atherosclerotic plaque—endothelial cells, platelets, smooth muscle cells, and tissue macrophages (derived from blood monocytes). Based on studies of diet-induced hypercholesterolaemia in primates, it is believed to be the endothelial cell which is the site where the lesion is initiated, but the actual cause has not been determined. There is increasing interest in the role of lipid oxidation in the initiation process. Oxidation of unsaturated fatty acids in LDL, caused by free radical attack, can be promoted by endothelial cells and by metals, *in vitro*. This results in changes in the lipoprotein that reduce its uptake by the usual LDL receptors on cells. However it is usually taken up by macrophages *in vitro* to form lipid-laden cells reminiscent of 'foam cells'. If this occurred in the body it could be the basis of the atherosclerotic plaque. An important event in the process is thought to be an alteration in the functional or structural barrier presented by the endothelial cell lining of the vessel, and it is probable that the properties of these cells are altered as a consequence of hyperlipidaemia. Monocytes can then enter the intima between endothelial cells and become lipid-filled; some remain here and this may further alter the cell properties. Smooth muscle cell proliferation and subsequent migration to the intima is also a focal and crucial process in atherosclerosis.

Experimental damage of arterial endothelium, exposing connective tissue to the blood, causes platelet activation and aggregation on the surface. Platelets then release thromboxanes (primarily thromboxane A) which increase platelet aggregation and lead to the contraction of smooth muscle cells within the arterial wall. Platelet aggregation and adherence to the damaged surface of the atherosclerotic plaque is intimately involved in thrombus formation. Platelets may be altered in hyperlipidaemia in a way that can promote aggregation. β-thromboglobulin, platelet factor 4, and other procoagulant materials are increased in the plasma of hyperlipidaemic subjects. Growth factors produced from the endothelial cells, monocytes, and the platelets, can cause proliferation and migration of the smooth muscle cells. *In vitro* evidence also suggests that LDL, particularly oxidized LDL, stimulates cell proliferation.

Oxidized LDL also has other properties which could promote atheroma and vascular occlusion if it is present in the vessel walls. These include binding to collagen, inhibition of endothelium-dependent relaxation, increased expression of adhesion molecules, and adverse effects on the coagulation pathways.

The type of atheromatous changes found in vessels of a man dying of premature vascular disease are shown in Fig. 3.1 and the possible sequence of events leading to the development of such lesions is shown diagrammatically in Fig. 3.2. The result of the process is an increase in the size of the atherosclerotic lesions, which may cause symptoms by reducing blood flow.

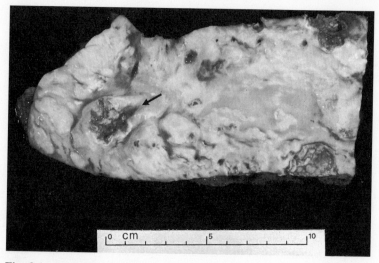

Fig. 3.1 Atheromatous aorta showing fibrous plaques. The lesion indicated has ulcerated.

The causes of myocardial infarction

Acute myocardial infarction nearly always occurs in people who already have significant coronary artery disease. The vulnerability of such individuals to actual infarction depends on a number of different factors. It is often the formation of thrombus in areas of vessels already significantly narrowed by atherosclerosis that causes the acute arterial occlusion resulting in the myocardial or cerebral infarction. This has been shown angiographically to be present in most cases of myocardial infarction and may account for the association between CHD events and plasma concentrations of fibrinogen and some clotting factors. The actual thrombotic incident may be precipitated by fissure of an athero-sclerotic plaque which would provide the acute stimulus to platelet aggregation and thrombus formation. It is also possible that less well understood factors contribute, such as coronary spasm.

Risk factors

A risk factor is a measurable parameter whose variance explains a pro-portion of the variance of the rate of the disease.

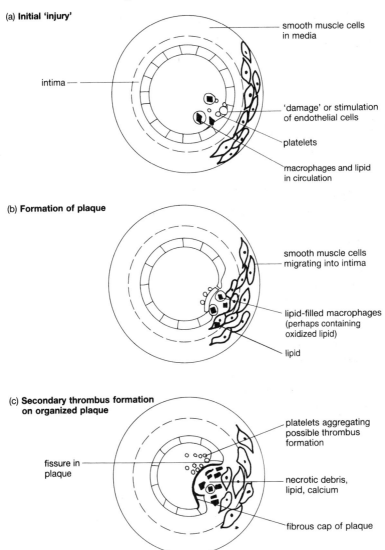

(a) **Initial 'injury'**

smooth muscle cells
in media

intima

'damage' or stimulation
of endothelial cells

platelets

macrophages and lipid
in circulation

(b) **Formation of plaque**

smooth muscle cells
migrating into intima

lipid-filled macrophages
(perhaps containing
oxidized lipid)

lipid

(c) **Secondary thrombus formation
on organized plaque**

platelets aggregating
possible thrombus
formation

fissure in
plaque

necrotic debris,
lipid, calcium

fibrous cap of plaque

Fig. 3.2 Schematic representation of the possible changes occurring in a
vessel to cause atheromatous lesions and potential vessel occlusion.

Risk factors for atherosclerosis and coronary heart disease

Age, sex, cigarette smoking, hypertension, hyperlipidaemia, diabetes, and obesity are the most important factors associated with the development of atherosclerotic disease. Most of the risk factors have a stronger effect in younger people. The relationship of CHD with hypertension and with plasma lipid levels is almost linear over a range of values.

Age and sex

Atherosclerosis of the coronary and cerebral circulation tends to occur later in life in women, but it increases with age in both sexes. The precise mechanism by which premenopausal women are protected against CHD is not understood, but the rate is much lower in young women than men of a comparable age. Women who undergo oophorectomy before the age of 35 have a relative risk of CHD of about seven times that of age-matched controls. CHD frequency increases rapidly after the menopause, but at no age does the rate exceed that of men.

Hyperlipidaemia

The risk of developing atherosclerotic heart disease is directly correlated with plasma cholesterol concentration and up to a third of the weight of atherosclerotic plaques is cholesterol. The mechanism by which cholesterol accumulates in the plaques is not clearly understood, but it appears to be derived from the plasma. This could cause an alteration in the cholesterol to phospholipid ratio in the membranes. Circulating lipoprotein, particularly LDL, can be detected in normal vessel walls in very low concentration. Altered LDL is also found in early atherosclerotic plaques. It is possible that if a breach occurs in the endothelium, due to physical or chemical damage, it would allow an influx of LDL into the intima. Lipoproteins could also be absorbed into the intimal connective tissue matrix and be taken up by cells of the arterial wall. High concentrations of LDL or VLDL may thus result in lipid accumulation in the vessel wall. The positive relationship between total and LDL cholesterol and triglyceride, and the inverse association between HDL cholesterol and CHD, were discussed in more detail in Chapter 2. HDL may be the strongest negative predictor of CHD in women.

People with hyperlipidaemia often have another risk factor for CHD. Identification and treatment of these factors is most important. It appears that raised plasma lipids enhance the damaging effects of other parameters. For example, in Japan hypertension is quite common, but CHD is relatively rare in those who eat the basic Japanese diet which is low in saturated fat. However, if they move to an area where they consume a diet high in saturated fat then their risk of developing CHD increases.

Raised $Lp_{(a)}$

$Lp_{(a)}$ is present in differing amounts in individuals, and high levels appear to be a risk factor for CHD and for stroke. Family studies and twin studies indicate that $Lp_{(a)}$ levels are highly heritable.

The mechanisms by which $Lp_{(a)}$ is atherogenic is unknown.

Cigarette smoking

Smoking is strongly related to cardiovascular disease in countries where CHD rates are high (Fig. 3.3). Large prospective studies have shown that men who smoke more than 20 cigarettes a day have three to four times the risk of dying from CHD than those who do not smoke. Furthermore, the relationship between smoking and CHD is linear. Smokers also have an increased risk of stroke and intermittent claudication. Sudden cardiac death is frequently the first clinical manifestation of CHD, and is three times more common than in non-smokers. Atherosclerotic changes found at post mortem correlate with smoking habits, and the association applies to changes in the aorta, the large coronary arteries, and the small intramyocardial arteries. Heavy cigarette smokers with high carboxyhaemoglobin levels have a particularly high risk of vascular disease, and may develop symptoms at an earlier stage of the disease because of the slightly lowered blood oxygen content. Cigarette smokers who undergo coronary artery bypass have a higher perioperative mortality than non-smokers. The mechanisms mediating the adverse effects of smoking may include increased platelet aggregability, increase in fibrinogen levels, increase in 'oxidative' stress, and a small effect on HDL cholesterol.

Figure 3.3 shows that the association of CHD with cigarette smoking is much less striking among Southern European men. Smoking more than

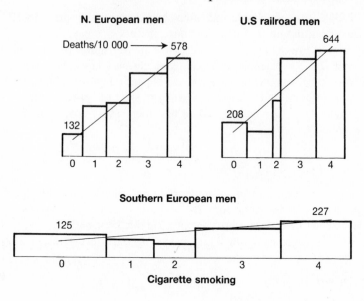

Fig. 3.3 Relationship of smoking and CHD deaths in different countries. (From Keys, A. (1980). *Seven countries. A multivariate analysis of death and coronary heart disease.* Harvard University Press.)

20 cigarettes per day among this group is associated with only a two-fold increase of fatal CHD compared with non-smokers. This group have a lower saturated fat intake and cholesterol level suggesting that the higher plasma lipids in the northern Europeans and Americans enhances the damaging effect of other risk factors. Again, in Japan, where both cigarette smoking and hypertension are common, but cholesterol levels are low, CHD occurs relatively infrequently.

Discontinuation of smoking causes a fall in the augmented risk to a normal range after two or three years.

Hypertension

A near linear association is found in high-risk populations between systolic and diastolic blood pressure and CHD. This applies at relatively low levels as well as elevated values. As with cholesterol it is difficult to identify a cut-off point associated with a particularly high risk. The

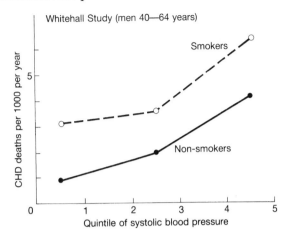

Fig. 3.4 Smoking and systolic blood pressure as risk factors for CHD. From the Whitehall study of British civil servants (Reid *et al.* (1976). *Lancet*, **ii**, 979–84).

Framingham Study showed that a systolic blood pressure greater than 160 mmHg or a diastolic greater than 95 mmHg carries a two- to three-fold increased risk of CHD, and an even greater risk of cerebral vascular disease. Treatment of patients with moderate hypertension seems to reduce the overall mortality, but this is mainly by reducing the incidence of strokes. The interactive relationship between risk factors—systolic blood pressure and smoking—is shown in Fig. 3.4

There is increasing interest in the metabolic associations of hypertension and how they contribute to CHD risk.

Obesity

Significant obesity confers an increased risk of CHD, but it is unclear to what extent this is an independent risk as obese people often have raised blood pressure, plasma glucose, and plasma lipids. Obesity is, however, common in many Western countries and whether its influence is secondary or not, obesity is a useful way of identifying those at increased CHD risk. In the large US Nurses' Health Study there was a strong association between body mass index (BMI) and the occurrence of myocardial infarction. An idea of the percentage of the population who are overweight (BMI > 25) and seriously overweight

Table 3.1   Men and women with BMI exceeding values indicative of CHD risk: data for New Zealand, Britain, and Australia

Age	Men			Women		
	25–34	35–49	50–64	25–34	35–49	50–64
New Zealand (1989)						
% BMI > 25	43	61	67	28	39	58
% BMI > 30	6	13	13	7	13	19
Britain (1987)						
% BMI > 25	36	52	62	27	40	52
% BMI > 30	6	11	9	6	11	10
Australia (1989)						
% BMI > 25	43	55	61	23	35	51
% BMI > 30	8	11	14	8	11	18

(BMI > 30) in some countries is given by Table 3.1. Central obesity appears to be particularly important with respect to CHD risk, and waist:hip ratio may be useful in characterizing this type of fat distribution.

Syndrome X

It has increasingly been recognized that there is a clinical and metabolic picture of insulin resistance, hypertension, and hypotriglycoidaemia, which may be associated with obesity, but not necessarily.

Diabetes or glucose intolerance

Individuals with diabetes or impaired glucose tolerance (as defined in Chapter 6) are at substantially increased risk of CHD, although the relationship with a single glucose measurement is less convincing. Women are particularly susceptible to the effects of diabetes. In diabetic women the usual protective effect of the female sex is lost. The presence of a high insulin level is also associated with the subsequent development of CHD. The precise mechanism by which diabetes increases the risk of CHD has not been established. However, lipid abnormalities are common and the triglyceride-rich lipoproteins may be more susceptible to oxidation by free radicals. Platelet aggregation may also be increased. It is not clear whether basement membrane abnormalities contribute.

Pre-existing CHD

The risk of subsequent coronary events is several times greater in people who have pre-existing CHD.

Exercise

Exercise is difficult to evaluate as an independent variable since those taking regular exercise are self-selected and exercise can affect other important variables. Nevertheless studies have shown that those involved in regular, heavy, physical work have a reduced risk of sudden death, and physical fitness is a predictor of CHD mortality in asymptomatic North American men. Those who engage in vigorous exercise in their leisure time also have a lower incidence of myocardial infarction than inactive individuals. In addition, people who take regular exercise appear to have a slightly lower risk of developing hypertension, and exercise can be of value in those attempting to lose weight. Regular vigorous exercise has been shown to increase HDL levels slightly.

Ethnic origin and psychosocial factors

People of Asian origin living in Britain have a higher CHD mortality than Caucasians. The mortality is higher than those living in their country of origin, perhaps reflecting the effects of genetic predisposition plus the acquisition of other factors while living in Britain. People from the Caribbean also have a high mortality from stroke and hypertensive disease, and New Zealand Maori have a higher incidence of CHD than non-Maori New Zealanders. Australian aborigines who eat a 'Western diet' have a very high incidence of obesity, diabetes, and CHD. Some authorities consider that they have a 'thrifty genotype' that was adapted to 'bush diet' conditions.

Mortality from CHD is higher overall in unskilled workers (social classes IV and V) than in the professional classes and the gap has widened in the last decade (Fig. 3.5). Mortality is also high in those who are unemployed, who constitute an increasing percentage of the population in many countries. This is partly accounted for by a different frequency of other risk factors in these groups.

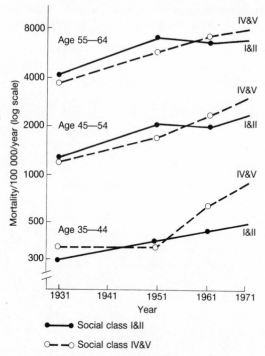

Fig. 3.5 Relationship between social class and CHD. (From Marmot *et al.* (1978). *British Medical Journal*, **ii**, 1109–12.)

There has been debate about the role of 'stress' in the development of CHD and about what constitutes stress as precise measures have proved elusive. In the Whitehall Study of British civil servants there was a stepwise inverse relationship between employment grade and CHD mortality. Those in the lower grades did tend to smoke more, had a higher mean blood pressure, less leisure-time physical activity, and a higher prevalence of diabetes and obesity, but it appeared that this did not account for the entire difference in CHD. Job characteristics such as 'lack of control' over the work and poor social support may be important. Longitudinal studies show the unemployed to have a 20 per cent higher mortality rate from CHD than the employed.

Personality factors

Some studies have indicated that people with a type-A behaviour (aggressive, ambitious, and restless, with an increased sense of time-urgency) have a greater risk of CHD and sudden death than those with a more passive type-B behaviour. This concept was devised in white Caucasian males and is difficult to evaluate. The relationship in this group may be partly related to other risk factors in some of the men with type-A behaviour. Of note is the apparent contradiction between this theory and the findings of studies such as the Whitehall Study, where type-A behaviour was commoner in those of higher grades yet they had a lower overall CHD mortality.

Clotting factors

The effects of the clotting factors were extensively studied in the Northwick Park Prospective Study. Factor VII coagulant activity and fibrinogen appear to be strongly related to the subsequent development of CHD and the predictive effect may be as strong as that of plasma cholesterol. Genetic factors may be important, but it is of interest that fibrinogen levels are increased by cigarette smoking and factor VIIc levels are related to the intake of saturated fat.

Deficiencies of particular proteins, such as protein S, may also account for an increased thrombotic tendency in some individuals.

Genetic factors

A tendency for CHD to run in families has been recognized for a long time. It was initially assumed that inherited forms of hyperlipidaemia and inherited factors in diabetes, and possibly hypertension, accounted for this finding. Several studies have now shown that the familial aggregation of CHD is not exclusively mediated by familial resemblance in plasma cholesterol and other classical risk factors. The risk related to a strong family history of CHD was demonstrated in the Framingham Study where analysis showed that the incidence of myocardial infarction in brothers was significantly related after the effects of cholesterol, blood pressure, and smoking had been controlled. It is possible that a tendency to hypercoagulability may be present in some of the families with an increased incidence of premature CHD and no obvious risk factors, but it is likely that there are a number of other important genetic factors. These may include factors such as Lp(a), which was not measured in the prospective studies. Recent advances in techniques in molecular biology are allowing investigation of some genetic factors which may be related to the development of premature CHD. Such techniques are likely to increase our understanding of the high degree of heritability of the disease.

Summary

Atherosclerosis is usually the basic pathology underlying the development of symptomatic CHD. There are a number of factors which appear to accelerate the development of atherosclerosis. Elevated plasma cholesterol is of major importance and it also appears to enhance the adverse effects of other risk factors.

4

Does lipid lowering reduce coronary heart disease risk?

Populations with low mean cholesterol levels have low rates of CHD and within high-risk populations there is a gradient of CHD risk with increasing levels of cholesterol. Studies on migrants show that the CHD risk of populations can be modified by changes in diet, blood cholesterol, and other environmental factors. When Japanese, who traditionally have a low risk of CHD, migrate to Hawaii or the USA they soon tend to acquire rates which approximate to those in the host country. On the other hand, Finns who live in Sweden, where CHD rates are relatively low, have appreciably lower rates than when living in their native Finland where CHD rates are among the highest in the world. Thus, it would be reasonable to assume that succeeding generations exposed to a way of life expected to be associated with reduced cardiovascular risk factors would have appreciably lower CHD rates. However it is also important to establish whether individual members of particular populations would benefit from making lifestyle changes or taking lipid-lowering medications. This chapter summarizes the clinical trials which have been performed to establish whether cholesterol lowering over a relatively short period of time can achieve a reduction in morbidity and mortality from CHD, or cause regression of atherosclerosis.

Effect of lipid-lowering treatment on angiographic change

A series of studies involving sequential coronary angiography has suggested that lipid lowering can produce regression of atherosclerosis over a relatively short time frame (1–5 years). The studies have included patients with a range of lipid disorders and the effects appear to be related to the extent of cholesterol lowering rather than the means by which it was achieved. Two recent studies serve as examples. The Lifestyle Heart Trial involved random allocation of 48 subjects to a 'usual care' group or an experimental group who received advice concerning a strict vegetarian diet (fat providing as little as 10 per cent total energy and carbohydrate 70–75 per cent total energy), smoking cessation, stress management training, and regular physical activity. Quantitative angiography after a year showed that in the experimental group the mean percentage diameter stenosis in the coronary arteries regressed from 40 per cent to 37 per cent in association with a 37 per cent fall in LDL-cholesterol, whereas among the controls there was progression from 42 per cent to 46 per cent. While the extent of the dietary intervention may limit application of the results, the findings provide an indication of the rapid benefits of appreciable reduction in LDL-C.

The STARS (St Thomas' Angiographic Regression Study) study involved computer-assisted assessment of coronary angiograms for quantifying atherosclerosis and contrasts between experimental and control groups which are more relevant to routine clinical practice. Ninety men with CHD and a plasma cholesterol greater than 6.5 mmol/l were randomized to receive usual care (UC), dietary advice (D), or diet and cholestyramine (DC). The diet was comparable to that usually recommended for such patients (saturated and total fat of 8–10 per cent and about 28 per cent total energy respectively, P:S ratio of 0.8–1.0). During the approximately 3-year follow-up period mean plasma cholesterol levels were 6.9 mmol/l (UC), 6.2 mmol/l (D), and 5.6 mmol/l (DC). The proportions of patients showing overall progression of coronary stenosis were 46 per cent (UC), 15 per cent (D), and 12 per cent (DC). The mean absolute width of the coronary segments increased significantly in DC and to some extent in D, the changes being significantly correlated with the LDL: HDL ratio. Thus there would seem to be little doubt that lipid lowering can favourably influence the pathological process underlying clinical CHD, but large scale clinical trials are necessary to determine the extent to which this benefit will be reflected in a reduction of clinical events.

Clinical trials of cholesterol lowering by diet and drugs

Most early studies of cholesterol lowering were aimed at modifying only one factor and the majority were too small to produce meaningful conclusions in terms of morbidity and mortality as the confidence intervals are very wide. Only a few studies warrant individual mention.

Los Angeles Veterans Administration Study

In this study, 846 male volunteers (aged 55–89) received either a 'control' diet (40 per cent energy from fat, mostly saturated, typical of the North American diets) or an 'experimental' diet (with half as much cholesterol and predominantly polyunsaturated vegetable oils replacing approximately two-thirds of the animal fat). As a result of skilled food technology the study was conducted under double-blind conditions. The follow-up period was eight years.

It was found that:

- cholesterol levels in the experimental group were 13 per cent lower
- deaths due solely to atherosclerotic events were appreciably reduced as compared with the controls (see Table 4.1)
- the beneficial effect of the cholesterol-lowering diet was most marked in those with initial high plasma cholesterol levels.

Deaths due to conditions other than CHD and from uncertain causes occurred more frequently in the experimental group, though no single cause predominated. The increase in non-cardiovascular mortality in the experimental group raised for the first time the suggestion that cholesterol lowering might be harmful in some respects despite the reduction in CHD.

Coronary drug project

A total of 8000 men with a history of myocardial infarction were randomized to five active treatments or placebo.

It was found that three of the therapies (conjugated oestrogens 2.5 mg and 5.0 mg daily and dextrothyroxine 6.0 mg daily) were associated with an excess mortality in comparison with placebo. Clofibrate (1.8 g daily) was associated with a non-significant reduction of CHD, and niacin (3 g daily) with a significant reduction in non-fatal myocardial infarction which persisted during a 15-year follow-up.

WHO collaborative trial of clofibrate

A total of 15 745 healthy men aged 30–59 were allocated to three groups on the basis of their cholesterol levels. Half of those in the

Table 4.1 Summary tabulation of deaths by category in the
Los Angeles Veterans Administration Study

Category	Number of cases	
	Control	Experimental
Due to acute atherosclerotic event (sole cause)	60	39
Mixed causes, including acute atherosclerotic event	10	9
Due to atherosclerotic complication without acute event	1	2
Mixed causes, including atherosclerotic complication with acute event	10	7
Other causes	71	85
Uncertain causes	25	32
Total	177	174

(From Dayton, S., *et al.* (1969). *Circulation*, **39**, suppl. 11, 1–63.)

upper third of the cholesterol distribution were randomly assigned to
clofibrate treatment (Group 1) and the other half to indistinguishable
olive oil capsules (Group 2). A second control group (Group 3), chosen
randomly from the lowest third of the cholesterol distribution, was also
given olive oil. The trial was carried out under double-blind conditions.

It was found that:

● during the five years of active therapy a 9 per cent reduction of
  cholesterol was achieved on clofibrate
● there was a significant reduction of major CHD in Group 1 compared
  with Group 2
● the difference between the two groups was due to cholesterol lowering
● men with the highest initial cholesterol, the greatest reduction during
  the trial, and those with other CHD risk factors, had the greatest
  reduction in non-fatal CHD.

There was, however, a significant increase in mortality in the clofibrate group. This was due to a variety of causes, with no particular disease (except for gallstones) predominating, and there was no relation between excess mortality and cholesterol reduction. The excess mortality in the clofibrate group did not continue after discontinuation of the drug, and may have related to effects of the particular drug, which is very seldom used now.

The initial hypothesis behind the trial was that reduction of plasma cholesterol would reduce the incidence of CHD; this was confirmed. Clofibrate therapy was merely the chosen method of reduction.

Lipid research clinics coronary primary prevention trial

This multicentre, randomized, double-blind study tested the efficacy of cholesterol lowering in reducing the risk of CHD in 3806 asymptomatic men with primary hypercholesterolaemia which had not responded to simple dietary management. The treatment group received the bile acid sequestrant cholestyramine and the control group received a placebo, for an average of 7.4 years.

The cholestyramine group experienced a mean reduction in total plasma and LDL cholesterol of 13.4 per cent and 20.3 per cent respectively.

In comparison with the placebo group there was:

- a 24 per cent reduction in fatal CHD
- a 19 per cent reduction in non-fatal myocardial infarction
- an appreciably reduced incidence rate for new positive exercise tests, angina, and coronary bypass surgery (Fig.4.1).

The reduction of CHD incidence in the cholestyramine group appeared to be mediated chiefly by the fall in total and LDL cholesterol.

Accidents and violence occurred more frequently (though not significantly so) in the cholestyramine group, but deaths from all other causes were similar in the two groups.

The Helsinki Heart Study

Inclusion in this study was based on the level of the non-HDL cholesterol (LDL plus VLDL cholesterol): 4081 men with a non-HDL cholesterol >5.2 mmol/l were randomized to receive gemfibrozil

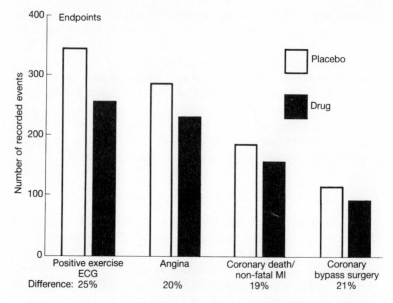

Fig. 4.1 Results of the Lipid Research Clinics Primary Prevention Trial.

600 mg b.d. or placebo for a five-year period. Gemfibrozil gave a mean reduction of 8 per cent for plasma cholesterol, 9 per cent for LDL cholesterol, and 40 per cent for plasma triglycerides. HDL cholesterol increased by about 11 per cent.

A difference in the incidence of cardiac disease between the two groups was seen after two years. The cumulative rate of cardiac endpoints at five years was 27 per 1000 in the gemfibrozil treated group and 44 per 1000 in the placebo group. The reduction in CHD in the treated group was 34 per cent.

Overall perspective of the clinical trials

As has already been indicated many of the individual studies (especially the smaller ones) are subject to a considerable margin of error. A series of meta-analyses has attempted to reduce this and provide an overall perspective. The first of these was carried out by Peto *et al.* (1987) who fitted confidence intervals to the differences in CHD rates between the control and experimental groups. Figure 4.2 shows the

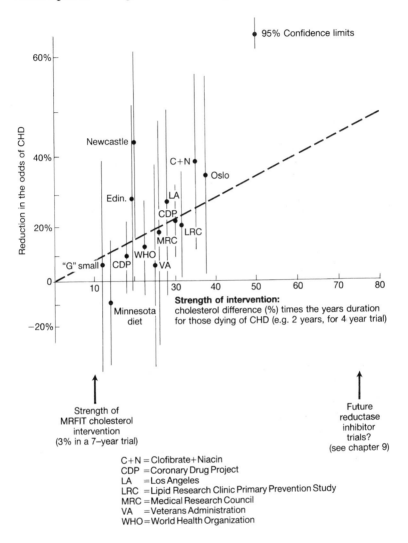

Fig. 4.2 CHD reduction versus strength of intervention in the unconfounded randomized trials. (Peto, R. *et al.*, reproduced with permission.)

drop in risk of CHD in the various trials in relation to achieved cholesterol lowering (presented as strength of intervention calculated by multiplying the cholesterol difference between experimental and control

Table 4.2   Overall estimates of effect on total CHD of a 'standard' 10 per cent cholesterol reduction in a four-year trial, using various lipid-lowering methods

	Number of trials	Estimated CHD reduction
Clofibrate	4	16% ± 5%
Niacin	2	14% ± 5%
Clofibrate and niacin	1	24% ± 9%
Bile acid sequestrants	5	15% ± 7%
Diet	8	13% ± 6%
All unconfounded randomized trials	20	16% ± 3%

groups by years duration). The association between the strength of intervention and reduction in CHD risk is impressive. On average each 1 per cent fall in cholesterol produces a 2 per cent reduction in CHD. The longer the trial has been continued, the more striking the beneficial effect. Furthermore a similar effect is apparent regardless of the means by which cholesterol lowering is achieved (Table 4.2).

More recent meta-analyses have concentrated on cardiovascular and other causes of mortality rather than on total cardiovascular events. Not surprisingly the results tend to depend to a considerable extent on the studies included. Several studies were carried out on institutionalized psychiatric patients. In the V.A. study the excessive number of non-cardiac deaths occurred in the group who were defined as non-compliant. In other studies the increase in non-cardiac mortality occurred after the active treatment had been stopped. In summary it is possible to draw the following conclusions with regard to mortality. First, the beneficial effect of cholesterol lowering is generally greater when considering non-fatal rather than fatal cardiovascular events. Second, in most studies, particularly those in which drugs have been used to lower cholesterol, the reduction in cardiovascular events has been offset by an increase in non-cardiac mortality, most notably deaths from accidents and violence (including suicide). There is no clear explanation for this observation which has not been consistent and in most individual studies not statistically significant. Mortality from non-cardiac causes has not been related to the extent of cholesterol lowering nor is it in keeping with the epidemiological evidence. On the other hand the benefit of cholesterol lowering on CHD is specific, highly statistically significant, proportional to the cholesterol-lowering achieved, and in keeping with the epidemiological evidence. Nevertheless the degree of uncertainty is such that it is generally considered appropriate to reserve drug therapy for those at particularly great risk of CHD because of a familial hyperlipidaemia, established CHD or coexistent risk factors because among them the benefit of cholesterol lowering is especially striking and likely to outweigh any conceivable adverse effects. In general these are not considered to be adverse effects of the sort of dietary changes currently recommended and the results of multifactorial intervention trials, in which attempts are made to alter diet and other risk factors present, are particularly encouraging.

Multiple risk factor intervention studies

European Collaborative Trial

A multicentre trial introduced health education into selected factories in four countries. Individuals in different factories were paired; one of each pair received education and the other acted as a control. The health education included advice on diet (aimed at cholesterol lowering and reduction of obesity), emphasized the importance of not smoking and of increased physical activity, and gave information on hypertension. In addition, men with a mean systolic blood pressure above 160 mmHg were started on antihypertensive drug therapy.

It was found that:

- only small net reductions in risk factors were achieved
- the reduction in overall CHD mortality was only 7.4 per cent.

Support that this represented more than just a chance improvement came from the results from individual centres. The UK had the least risk factor reduction and showed no evidence of a fall in CHD incidence. Belgium and Italy produced the greatest reduction in risk factors and greater changes in CHD incidence: for example, in Belgium, there was a highly significant 24 per cent reduction in CHD.

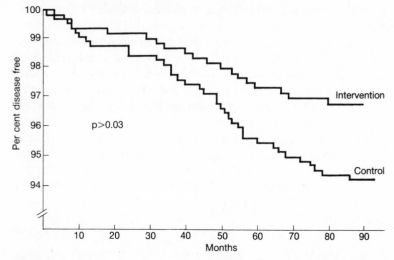

Fig. 4.3 Life table analysis of CHD (fatal and non-fatal myocardial infarction and sudden death) in intervention and control groups. The Oslo Study. (From Hjermann, I. *et al.* (1981). *Lancet*, **ii**, 1303–10.)

Oslo Trial

In the Oslo Trial, men at high risk of CHD (as a result of smoking or having a cholesterol level in the range of 7.5–9.8 mmol/l) were divided into two groups; half received intensive dietary education and advice to stop smoking, the other half served as a control group.

It was found that:

- a reduction (31 versus 57 per 1000 over a five-year period) in total coronary events occurred (see Fig. 4.3) in association with a 13 per cent fall in cholesterol and a 65 per cent reduction in tobacco consumption
- there was a significant improvement in total mortality in the treated groups, and no significant differences between the two groups for non-cardiac causes of death.

Detailed statistical analysis suggests that approximately 60 per cent of the CHD reduction can be attributed to serum cholesterol change and 25 per cent to smoking reduction.

Multiple risk factor intervention trial (MRFIT)

Over 24 000 men at risk were chosen on the basis of plasma cholesterol level and smoking (similar to the Oslo study) and of high blood pressure. Intervention against these three risk factors for six years in the 'special intervention' group was compared with the control group randomized to 'usual care'. The results are shown below.

	Intervention group	Control group
Smoking	Reduction of 50 per cent	Reduction of 29 per cent
Diastolic B.P.	Fall of 10.5 mm Hg	Fall of 7.3 mm Hg
Serum cholesterol	Fall of 5 per cent	Fall of 3 per cent

The changes in the control group were presumed to result from the widespread coronary prevention education in the USA.

Clearly, a trial which achieves a reduction in plasma cholesterol in the intervention group only 2 per cent greater than the control group cannot be used to determine whether a reduction in plasma cholesterol will lead to a reduction in CHD incidence. Furthermore, over the study period, CHD mortality in the USA declined by 25 per cent. As a result of this, and of the risk-factor reduction in controls as well as the intervention group, both groups had lower than predicted mortality and there were no significant differences between the groups during the first six years.

However, after 10 years of follow-up, mortality rates from CHD were 10.6 per cent lower in the 'special care' than in the 'usual care' group. There was also a trend towards lower overall mortality as well as lower death rates from cancer and violence in the intervention group. The MRFIT underlines the near impossibility of achieving an appropriate control group now that many people are aware of coronary risk factors and their consequences. Further large multifactorial intervention trials are unlikely to be carried out, but perhaps this does not matter too much since there is widespread agreement regarding the potential benefit of lifestyle change particularly in high risk individuals.

Summary

Cholesterol lowering by diet or drugs reduces the risk of coronary events in proportion to the cholesterol lowering achieved. The benefits are primarily in terms of reducing premature morbidity from CHD and reinfarction and are seen even when treatment is initiated in middle age. While high risk individuals may experience prolongation of life there is no impressive evidence for an overall increase in life expectancy. This may occur in future generations who have reduced lifetime exposure to lifestyle-related cardiovascular risk factors. There is no evidence of any risks associated with lifestyle changes. However, the unresolved issue concerning possible untoward effects of some drug treatments on non-cardiac mortality lead to the recommendation that drug therapy should be reserved for those at particularly high CHD risk in whom lifestyle measures have not succeeded in reducing lipid levels, since among them the benefits are likely to outweigh any possible risks.

Section II

Hyperlipidaemia: diagnosis and management

5

Hyperlipidaemia: diagnosis and assessment

The presence of raised plasma lipids alone seldom causes any symptoms or physical signs until the secondary pathologies of atherosclerosis or pancreatitis occur. Yet hyperlipidaemia, which poses a long-term threat to health, is very common. As discussed in other sections, a reduction in plasma cholesterol appears to be effective in reducing the incidence of CHD, both in individuals and in populations.

The data in Chapter 2 shows that it is impossible to identify thresholds for the unequivocal definition of hyperlipidaemia as there is a continuous gradient of risk associated with increasing plasma cholesterol levels (Fig. 5.1). For this reason 'action limits' are based to some extent on the practical consideration that it would be impossible to deal individually with everyone at some degree of risk. The levels below are based on those suggested by the European Atherosclerosis Society.

Cholesterol level (mmol/l)

Statistical reference range	Desirable	At some CHD risk	Identify for individual care
3.9–7.8	<5.2	5.2–6.5	>6.5

We would like to emphasize that these levels are suggested in the realization that those identified for individual care will need attention and follow-up, even though most will be symptom free. If universal screening were to be introduced then about a quarter of the adult population would currently be in this category, which is an awesome prospect. This would include those with severe inherited forms of hyperlipidaemia who have an exceptionally high risk of CHD and some whose risk of a first or further cardiovascular event is high because they already have CHD or other cardiovascular risk factors. Others in this

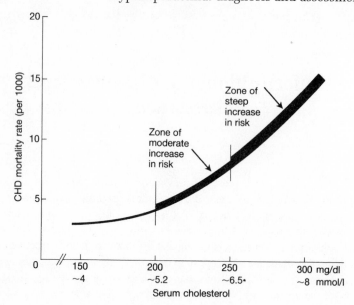

Fig. 5.1 CHD mortality rate in six years (MRFIT (1982), 356 222 men, aged 35–57).

category who have no other risk factors will be at a lesser degree of risk. When hyperlipidaemia is not due to a primary genetic disorder or secondary to another condition it is usually a consequence of a high-fat diet or obesity interacting with poorly defined genetic factors (polygenic hyperlipidaemia). The successful implementation of a population dietary strategy (Chapter 11) would greatly reduce the number of people with hyperlipidaemia and many others identified would respond to more specific dietary advice and not require drug treatment.

Much less information is available concerning desirable and 'at risk' plasma triglyceride levels. The European Atherosclerosis Society has suggested individual consideration of levels above 2.3 mmol/l. However, at present for most practical purposes we suggest that, in the presence of desirable levels of cholesterol, especially if LDL and HDL levels are satisfactory, people should only be identified for individual follow-up if triglycerides are greater than 3 mmol/l. We currently suggest that the initial diagnosis of hyperlipidaemia is based on a total cholesterol concentration greater than 6.5 mmol/l in adults and/or a fasting triglyceride concentration greater than 3 mmol/l.

It is important that ways be found to identify individuals with hyperlipidaemia, preferably before any symptoms of CHD develop. The most direct method would be to set up a specific service to screen the entire population in the age group 25–60 years, in conjunction with screening for other risk factors such as smoking and hypertension. In the absence of this comprehensive approach being considered feasible or even desirable it is important to emphasize measurement of blood lipids in groups of people who are likely to be at particular risk of hyperlipidaemia and/or its adverse effects.

The circumstances under which lipid measurements should always be made include:

(1) people with proven CHD or other manifestations of atherosclerosis, especially when these develop at a young age (less than 55);
(2) relatives of people who develop CHD below the age of 55 or are themselves hyperlipidaemic;
(3) people with a disease which may secondarily raise blood lipids, such as diabetes, hypothyroidism, nephrotic syndrome, and severe obesity (BMI> 30);
(4) people with stigmata of severe hyperlipidaemia such as xanthomas and early corneal arcus;
(5) people with pancreatitis;
(6) people with another CHD risk factor such as hypertension.

If hyperlipidaemia is suspected, a fasting blood sample should be taken and cholesterol and triglyceride levels measured. The results are then interpreted in the light of the patient's medical history, drug history, family history, diet, and age. The patient should also have a physical examination, particularly looking for signs of lipid deposition—notably xanthelasma, corneal arcus, tendon xanthomas, and eruptive xanthomas.

This assessment process can be understood as dividing those with raised lipids into four groups:

1. A large number of people with hyperlipidaemia; as many as a third of the population in some countries, notably the UK and New Zealand. In this group the hyperlipidaemia is the result of a high-fat diet in susceptible individuals, which is sometimes accentuated by obesity or a mild degree of inefficiency in lipoprotein clearance. Most of these people will respond readily to a reduction in dietary fat intake to 'sensible' levels (see p. 80). Dietary management is thus the mainstay of their treatment. Drug therapy has no place in their management.

2. People with an underlying illness, either known or covert, which provokes an increase in plasma lipid levels, which may be mild or sometimes very severe. The cause of this secondary hyperlipidaemia must be identified (see Chapter 6). These patients sometimes respond to dietary management, but usually the causative illness must be effectively treated before the levels of the blood lipids fall. Occasionally the illness cannot be treated and a specific lipid-lowering diet and drugs have to be considered.

3. A group of people, maybe 1 per cent of the population, with a severe primary disorder of lipid metabolism caused by a major genetic defect (see Chapter 7). The hyperlipidaemia is usually severe and the response to simple dietary change is combined with drug treatment, and the approach should be aggressive once the diagnosis is made.

4. People with primary hyperlipidaemia which does not respond to dietary management and lifestyle changes, but who do not have any obvious family history, or an obviously identifiable biochemical defect. At present they are often said to have 'common hyperlipidaemia', and no doubt future research will delineate a number of different aetiologies in this group.

Figure 5.2 gives a simple outline of the suggested protocol for the assessment and diagnosis of a patient with raised blood lipids. Chapters 6 and 7 discuss the presentation and management of the secondary and primary hyperlipidaemias.

Secondary hyperlipidaemia (see Chapter 6) must be excluded at an early stage and appropriate treatment given. Dietary modification (see Chapter 8) should be recommended to all people with primary hyperlipidaemia. Those who do not respond to simple dietary advice require further investigation in order to establish a more precise diagnosis (see Chapter 7) and to decide upon appropriate drug therapy (see Chapter 9). This therapy will depend on a total assessment of CHD risk.

Laboratory investigation of hyperlipidaemia

Measurement of plasma cholesterol and triglyceride concentrations

Points to consider:

1. Plasma cholesterol levels tend to increase with age, and are lower in children than in adults.

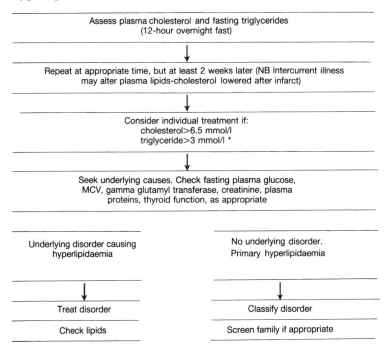

Fig. 5.2 Plan of investigation of people with hyperlipidaemia.

2. Slightly different values may be obtained when analyses are performed in different laboratories as standardization is difficult. Values given in subsequent discussion are for general guidance. It is sensible for serial measurements to be performed in one laboratory.

3. A myocardial infarction is often the event which causes the doctor to measure plasma lipids. Plasma lipids are affected by this, and other, severe illnesses. Plasma cholesterol often starts to fall about 24 hours after a myocardial infarct, and may remain at a reduced

level for up to two months. Plasma triglycerides may rise or, occasionally, fall.

4. Plasma cholesterol changes very slightly during the day, but the change in relation to meals is not noticeable. In contrast, plasma triglyceride concentrations are greatly affected by food intake, and specimens should be taken when patients are fasted.

5. It is important to repeat lipid measurements on more than one occasion before making management decisions.

Table 5.1   Possible effects of marked lipaemia on routine biochemical estimations

Analysis	Effect of lipaemia
Electrolytes	Lipids occupy space therefore interfere with the results of electrolyte determinations on flame photometers. Interference is less on an ion-specific electrode.
Liver enzymes including aspartate transminase	Results may be inaccurate, particularly estimations that involve kinetic enzymic assays, because of high 'blank'.
Amylase	May be falsely low by some methods.
Calcium	Measurement by fluorescence method may be low due to 'quenching'.
Blood gases	Interference depends on analyser (see manufacturer's information). Wash solution should be put through analyser after lipaemic samples to prevent accumulation of lipid on the electrode membrane.
Platelet count	On some counters lipid particles may be counted as platelets.

Note Fat emulsions given in parenteral nutrition may also cause lipaemia. It is wise to take blood 4–6 hours after lipid infusion to allow clearance.

6. Very high lipid levels may cause interference with other laboratory tests (Table 5.1).

When investigating the possibility of hyperlipidaemia in a patient as part of a routine screening procedure the total cholesterol and fasting triglyceride concentrations are the initial investigations. Consideration of the results together with information about the patients such as their history, physical signs, and their family history then usually allows a tentative diagnosis to be made. Measurement of HDL cholesterol and calculation of LDL may then be appropriate when the result is expected to affect the diagnosis or the decision on treatment. In the current financial climate it would seem a better use of resources to measure total cholesterol in more patients rather than performing lipoprotein fractions as the initial screening procedure. In people with CHD, a strong family history of CHD, or diabetes, however, the full fasting lipid profile should be obtained as the initial measurement.

Lipid concentrations in children

Knowledge about the plasma cholesterol and triglyceride concentrations which should be regarded as healthy for children is still imperfect. The largest epidemiological studies have been made in the USA. The statistically 'normal' values found in the Bogalusa Heart Study are shown in Table 5.2. It must, however, be remembered that in line with the situation in adults, those values probably do not represent healthy values, as many children in the Western world consume large quantities of saturated fat.

Table 5.2 Lipid levels in children — mean (5th, 95th centile)

Age	Total cholesterol (mmol/l)	HDL cholesterol (mmol/l)	Triglyceride (mmol/l)
Newborn (Cord blood)	1.8 (1.1, 2.1)	0.9 (0.3, 1.5)	0.4 (0.1, 0.9)
6 months	3.4 (2.3, 4.9)	1.3 (0.6, 2.2)	1.0 (0.6, 1.9)
1 year	3.9 (2.5, 4.9)	1.3 (0.6, 2.2)	0.9 (0.5, 1.8)
2–14 years	4.1 (3.1, 5.4)	1.7 (0.8, 2.6)	0.7 (0.4, 1.4)

Up to the age of five boys and girls have similar levels, but between five and 13 girls tend to have higher LDL and triglyceride levels. After puberty, the LDL levels rise in boys and their HDL levels become lower than those of girls, which is the situation in adults. When screening young children for hyperlipidaemia, measurement of the lipoprotein fractions is often needed and the results are best interpreted by someone with experience. Some people in the US advocate the screening of all children, but in our opinion measurement of blood lipids in children is only indicated in the presence of a family history of familial hyperlipidaemia or premature CHD.

Laboratory measurements

Cholesterol and triglyceride levels are measured enzymatically in most laboratories. Cholesterol measures on serum are 3–5 per cent higher than those on plasma.

Observation of serum or plasma stored overnight at 4 °C for opalescence (which indicates excess very low or intermediate density lipoprotein) or a creamy upper level of chylomicrons may be helpful.

Measurement of HDL cholesterol is generally appropriate as this is a determinant of risk and is particularly important in some people, such as diabetics, to delineate the lipid disorder. The various lipoproteins can be separated by a number of techniques including ultracentrifugation and chemical precipitation. The most commonly used methodology is the chemical precipitation of VLDL and LDL, and measurement of the HDL cholesterol left in the supernatant. If triglyceride levels (reflecting VLDL) are normal, then LDL constitutes most of the difference between the total and the HDL cholesterol. Some authors believe that the ratios of the various lipoproteins correlate well with CHD risk, but they may sometimes prove misleading. For example, incorrect risk assessment may be made if the total cholesterol/HDL cholesterol ratio is used without also measuring the triglycerides and estimating the LDL cholesterol.

$$\text{LDL cholesterol} = \text{total cholesterol} - \text{HDL cholesterol} - \frac{\text{triglyceride}}{2.3} \text{ (mmol/l)}$$

This can only be used if the plasma triglyceride concentration is below 4.5 mmol/l (400 mg/dL). Some laboratories calculate 'risk scores' from two or more results. It is important that people are aware of how these scores are calculated and the fact that they may be misleading in some cases. Lipoprotein electrophoresis is not generally helpful, although it is occasionally performed to examine for the presence of a broad B band. Measurement of lipoprotein lipase is complex, and only performed in a few specialized laboratories, but it may help in the diagnosis of selected cases of severe hypertriglyceridaemia.

Many of the apolipoproteins can now be measured by immunological methods and isoelectric focusing. Their use is now quite common in research studies and the usefulness of these measurements in clinical practice is under investigation. Some small retrospective studies have shown good correlation between apo B and apo B/apo A1 and CHD. There is, however, less prospective data or information from large studies such as that which exists for cholesterol and the lipoprotein fractions. Lp(a) can be measured by a number of techniques, and assay kits are available. Lp(a) and apoprotein determinations are being used in some centres and in research studies. Their likely value in routine practice needs assessment.

When considering laboratory analysis it is worth noting that severe hyperlipidaemia may cause problems in the determination of some routine blood and plasma analyses. This may sometimes cause difficulty in determining the underlying cause of some cases of severe secondary hyperlipidaemia, and in the biochemical investigation of concurrent diseases. Some of the problems which may be encountered are shown in Table 5.1. Of particular note is the fact that some types of assay for amylase activity are upset by a very high triglyceride level. This may cause a low result and a missed diagnosis of pancreatitis, which may in fact have resulted from the lipid abnormality.

Summary

There is no universal consensus concerning the most appropriate lipid measurements for routine clinical practice. Most laboratories measure cholesterol, triglyceride, and HDL cholesterol on a fasting blood sample and may also present a calculated measurement for LDL cholesterol provided triglyceride levels are not elevated (i.e. greater than 4.5 mmol/l). Measurements of Lp(a), apo B, and apo A_1 are increasingly being made when it is considered to be necessary to determine more precisely the lipoprotein mediated risk of CHD. In very selected hyperlipidaemic patients the lipoprotein profile may be further characterized after ultracentrifugation.

These measurements are increasingly, and appropriately, being considered together with other non-lipid risk factors in order to determine the absolute risk of CHD. Management of individuals with particular lipid levels may thus differ according to the assessment of overall CHD risk.

6

Secondary hyperlipidaemia

Diagnosis of secondary hyperlipidaemia

The first step in the management of a patient with hyperlipidaemia is to consider the possibility of an underlying cause, as lipid metabolism is altered in a number of physiological and pathological conditions. Secondary hyperlipidaemia, particularly due to obesity and a diet high in saturated fat, is common. Important causes of secondary hyperlipidaemia are shown in Table 6.1, together with the lipid changes which they tend to cause.

These conditions can usually be diagnosed by a full history and clinical examination, drug history, and determination of fasting plasma glucose, mean corpuscular cell volume, gamma glutamyl transpeptidase, thyroid, renal, and liver function tests, as considered necess-

Table 6.1 Conditions which may cause secondary hyperlipidaemia

Condition	Plasma cholesterol	Plasma triglycerides
Diabetes mellitus	(↑)	↑↑
Hypothyroidism	↑↑	↑
Excess alcohol intake		↑↑
Obesity	↑	↑
Nephrotic syndrome	↑↑	(↑)
Pregnancy	↑	
Biliary obstruction	↑	
Myeloma	↑	↑
Acute intermittent porphyria	↑	
Drugs—thiazides		↑
β blockers		↑
steroids	↑	↑
oral contraceptives		↑

ary. The response to the drugs mentioned may be general or idiosyncratic and a trial of exclusion or alternate medication may sometimes be appropriate. The effects of drug treatments are dealt with in Chapter 10. If a hyperlipidaemia is secondary then treatment of the underlying cause is usually associated with a reduction in lipid levels.

In children, noteworthy causes of secondary hyperlipidaemia include diabetes mellitus, hypothyroidism, idiopathic hypercalcaemia, and glycogen storage disease types I and III. Lipid levels rise in the second half of pregnancy.

Diabetes

A significant number of people with diabetes have quantitative and qualitative abnormalities of lipoproteins and changes in haemostatic parameters which may tend to increase coagulation. In type I diabetes, triglyceride levels are frequently elevated when control is not optimal. When control is good, LDL and HDL levels are usually similar to the non-diabetic population. HDL may even be higher, but its composition is altered in a way that may affect its function. Other abnormalities of lipoprotein composition can be seen, even in patients with normal cholesterol. Hyperlipidaemia is partly explained by the important role of insulin in both the catabolism of triglyceride-rich lipoproteins, and in LDL receptor activity. Insulin is necessary for the normal activity of lipoprotein lipase, and in the insulin deficiency of severe, uncontrolled diabetes mellitus the effect is of an acquired lipoprotein lipase deficiency resulting in markedly raised plasma triglyceride levels. This can occasionally cause the appearance of eruptive xanthomas (Fig. 6.1), hepatomegaly and lipaemia retinalis. Repletion of insulin restores lipoprotein lipase activity; the triglyceride levels fall and any eruptive xanthomas disappear.

In poorly controlled type I diabetes or in type II diabetes there is also a reduction in the peripheral use of glucose. Triglyceride in fat stores is broken down and fatty acids are released into the plasma; some are used by muscle, but a significant rise in blood levels may occur. Increased fatty acid mobilization leads to enhanced VLDL triglyceride secretion from the liver. Metabolism of the fatty acids also results in the formation of ketone bodies.

In type II diabetes, non-insulin-dependent diabetes, lipid abnormalities are very common (even when blood glucose control is fair or good). The usual pattern is a raised VLDL and triglycerides, for the

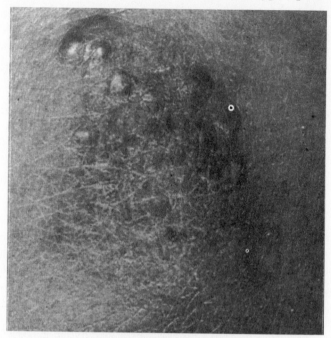

Fig. 6.1 Eruptive xanthomas.

reasons documented above. LDL levels may be normal but the LDL composition is usually abnormal. LDL is triglyceride rich and may be more susceptible to oxidation. Levels of HDL, particularly HDL2, are also often low. These abnormalities, together with alterations in platelet aggregation, clotting factors, and increased 'oxidative stress' associated with infection or ischaemia, may be responsible for the very high risk of CHD. Coexistent hypertension will accentuate this.

The advent of renal disease increases the risk of macrovascular disease to about 10–12 times that of age-matched non-diabetic controls. LDL cholesterol seems to be the most important factor associating with CHD in diabetic men, but HDL and apo AI may also be important in women, as may triglycerides in non-insulin-dependent diabetic women.

Dietary and lifestyle measures and optimization of glucose control partly improve the risk factor profile, but no randomized controlled trial has tested the effect on CHD.

Glucose intolerance and obesity

The adapted WHO criteria for the diagnosis of glucose intolerance are given in Table 6.2.

In the obese patient with mild glucose intolerance, hyperlipidaemia may be due to triglyceride and VLDL overproduction. These patients often have relatively high insulin levels, and several studies have

Table 6.2 Diagnosis of diabetes mellitus and impaired glucose tolerance. Based on the recommendations of the European Diabetes Epidemiology Study Group concerning the second report of the WHO Expert Committee. Diagnostic values for oral glucose tolerance test under standard conditions, using a load of 75 g glucose in 250–350 ml of water for adults, and of 1.75 g/kg body weight (to a maximum of 75 g) for children, and specific enzymatic glucose assay. Two classes of response are identified—diabetes mellitus and impaired glucose tolerance.

	Glucose concentration (mmol/l)		
	Venous whole blood	Capillary whole blood	Venous plasma
Diabetes mellitus			
Fasting and/or	≥6.7	≥6.7	≥7.8
2 hours after glucose load	≥10.0	≥11.0	≥11.1
Impaired glucose tolerance			
Fasting and	<6.7	<6.7	<7.8
2 hours after glucose load	6.7–9.9	7.8–11.0	7.8–11.0

The WHO Expert Committee recommended the following procedure for diagnosis:
1. If symptoms of diabetes are present, perform random or fasting blood glucose measurement. In adults, random venous or plasma values of 11 mmol/l or more or fasting values of 8 mmol/l or more are diagnostic. Random values below 8 mmol/l and fasting values below 6 mmol/l exclude the diagnosis.
2. If results are equivocal, measure blood glucose concentration two hours after 75 g of glucose taken orally after an overnight fast. Two-hour venous plasma glucose values of 11 mmol/l or more are diagnostic of diabetes. Values below 8 mmol/l are normal and those in the range 8–11 mmol/l are termed impaired glucose tolerance.

shown a relationship between plasma triglyceride and raised immuno-reactive insulin.

Hypothyroidism results in a rise in circulating LDL and total choles-terol levels. It may also cause hypertriglyceridaemia because of the reduc-tion in hepatic lipase activity, despite the fact that the supply of fatty acids to the liver is less due to reduced triglyceride breakdown in adipose tissue. Hypothyroidism may also result in a marked hyperlipidaemia if it occurs in genetically disposed people (see remnant hyperlipidaemia, Chapter 7). An effect on lipid levels may occur when the biochemical abnormalities are only mild and the person asymptomatic. There is usually a rapid fall in lipid levels in response to treatment with thyroxine.

Chronic renal failure

Raised levels of plasma triglycerides, or of triglycerides, LDL, and IDL cholesterol, may occur in chronic renal failure. This may be due to the reduced activity of hepatic lipase and lipoprotein lipase. VLDL produc-tion may also be increased and the composition of the lipoproteins abnormal. HDL levels tend to be low. Cardiovascular disease is one of the most frequent complications in patients with renal failure, and hyperlipidaemia may be an important risk factor in these patients. There is also concern that the lipid abnormalities may cause ongoing glomerular damage and glomerulosclerosis irrespective of the initial cause of the renal problem.

Haemodialysis and chronic ambulatory peritoneal dialysis do not usually improve the lipid abnormalities: in fact they often continue to deteriorate. The lipoprotein abnormalities may disappear after success-ful renal transplantation, although changes may persist if the patient has to remain on high doses of corticosteroids, because they reduce lipo-protein lipase activity.

Liver disease

Severe liver disease is accompanied by various disorders of lipid metabolism. Esterification of cholesterol is low because of reduced activity of the responsible enzyme. The lipoproteins often have an abnormal composition—and the abnormal lipoprotein X may be found. Raised plasma triglycerides are probably caused by low hepatic tri-glyceride lipase activity, but a triglyceride-rich LDL fraction may also contribute. HDL levels are often low.

All these changes are usually fully reversible and seem to be parameters indicating the degree of disturbance of liver function during inflammatory liver disease. Underlying alcohol abuse must be considered as this is notoriously under reported.

Alcohol excess   Alcohol causes a rise in plasma triglycerides primarily by inhibiting fatty acid activation and increasing fatty acid synthesis in the liver. VLDL output from the liver goes up. The amount of alcohol required to cause a significant rise in plasma levels depends on the individual—15–20 units per week may be enough in a susceptible person. The lipid levels often fluctuate. Some people can develop severe hypertriglyceridaemia and even chylomicronaemia after excessive alcohol intake. Pancreatitis can occur as a serious complication in such individuals where plasma triglyceride levels exceed 20 mmol/l. A marked fall in triglycerides and VLDL, and in body weight, can occur in response to abstinence.

Nephrotic syndrome

The causes of the hyperlipidaemia which often occur in this condition are unclear. In nephrotic syndrome there is an increase in hepatic protein synthesis as a response to the high urinary losses. Over production of the lipoproteins VLDL, and probably LDL, also seems to occur and the plasma levels are usually raised. HDL cholesterol and apo A1 levels may be very low if urinary losses are high. It is of note that it is the HDL subfraction, HDL2 (which is inversely related to CHD risk), which is particularly reduced. Another suggested mechanism for the lipoprotein changes is that hypoalbuminaemia causes fatty acids to bind to low affinity sites and increases fatty acid uptake by tissues including the liver, and this may increase VLDL synthesis. A further possibility is that hypoalbuminaemia causes an increase in apoprotein B synthesis.

It is not clear whether the CHD risk associated with secondary hyperlipidaemia is as high as might be expected considering the lipid levels. One factor which could be expected to explain a different risk from the inherited primary conditions is the duration of the hyperlipidaemia, which is generally shorter. Pancreatitis is, however, a significant risk in secondary hypertriglyceridaemia as in the primary conditions.

A plan for the identification of secondary hyperlipidaemia is shown in Fig. 6.2. For many of the conditions causing secondary hyperlipidaemia, such as hypothyroidism, effective treatment of the condition results in a reduction in plasma lipid levels.The response should, however, be checked because primary hyperlipidaemia is common and

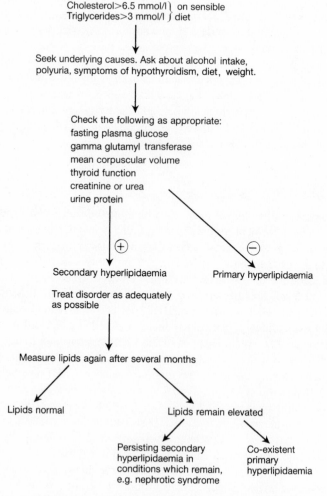

Fig. 6.2 Schematic diagram of investigations which should be considered in patients with hyperlipidaemia.

people may have this as well. In secondary cases, where treatment of the underlying condition is not possible or does not result in a reduction of lipid, as in some renal disorders, then specific treatment to lower the lipid levels may be necessary. In these cases the management required may be different from that which would usually be prescribed. For example, the diet advised for a patient with nephrotic syndrome and severe hyperlipidaemia will need to be specially designed for the individual patient. Consideration of drug treatment will also need to take into account the metabolism of the drug in the particular disease, for example bezafibrate must be given in reduced doses if it is used in patients with renal impairment.

Summary

Identification of secondary hyperlipidaemia is the first step in the assessment of any lipid abnormality. Conditions such as hypo-thyroidism and alcohol excess, which require specific treatment in their own right, may be identified because of the finding of hyperlipidaemia. Measurement of plasma lipids is also important in people with diabetes as they are at particular risk of developing CHD and other vascular complications.

7

Primary hyperlipidaemia

Once secondary hyperlipidaemia has been excluded, then characterization of the disorder is needed. A precise diagnosis is essential since these disorders have major implications concerning prognosis, genetic counselling, and lifelong diet and drug treatment.

Several classifications have been suggested for the primary hyperlipidaemias. The simplified genetic metabolic classification given in Table 7.1, based on that introduced by Goldstein *et al.*, is clinically more relevant than the World Health Organization (Fredrickson) classification based on the patterns seen on lipoprotein electrophoresis, as these are not specific to disease entities.

The distinct genetic conditions which are currently recognized are described in this chapter. It is likely that as our knowledge increases further groups will be delineated. At present those who have primary hyperlipidaemia, but do not obviously fit a condition described, are usually said to have 'common' hyperlipidaemia.

Familial hypercholesterolaemia

In this disorder there is a high concentration of LDL and total cholesterol in the circulation because of an inherited defect of LDL metabolism. The defect is usually a marked reduction in the number of the high-affinity LDL receptors on the surface of cells, which results in less LDL being removed from the circulation, but other defects such as functionally defective receptors and reduced receptor binding may give a similar picture. The increasing use of molecular biological techniques is revealing increasing numbers of defects responsible for these effects.

Familial hypercholesterolaemia (FH) is inherited in an autosomal dominant manner and is one of the commonest inherited conditions. In Britain, and a number of other countries, it is estimated that at least 1 in

Table 7.1   The Goldstein classification of primary
hyperlipidaemias

Characteristics of primary hyperlipidaemia [1]				↑ = raised; ↑↑= markedly raised; N = Normal	
	Atherosclerosis risk	Xanthomas	Inheritance	Relative prevalence	Lipid abnormalities	WHO type
Familial hypercholesterolaemia					
	+++	Tendon	Autosomal dominant	++	Cholesterol and LDL ↑↑ Triglyceride N or slightly ↑	IIa, occasionally IIb
Familial combined hyperlipidaemia					
	++	–	?	+++	Cholesterol and LDL↑ Triglyceride and VLDL ↑	IIb. occasionally IIa and IV
Remnant hyperlipoproteinaemia (broad beta)					
	++	Tuboeruptive palmar	Apo EIII deficiency and other factors	+	Cholesterol ↑↑ Triglycelride ↑↑ IDL ↑	III
Familial hypertriglyceridaemia					
Excessive synthesis	?	Eruptive	Probably autosomal dominant	+	Triglyceride and VLDL ↑↑ Chylomicrons ↑	IV. V
Lipoprotein lipase/apo CII deficiency	?	Eruptive	Probably recessive	rare	Triglyceride ↑↑ Chylomicrons ↑↑ VLDL ≠	I, V
Common hypercholesterolaemia					
	+		Polygenic	++++	Cholesterol and LDL ↑	IIa

[1]Adapted from Lewis B. Disorder of lipid transport in The Oxford textbook of medicine. Weatherall DJ Ledingham JGG. Warrell DA. eds. Oxford; Oxford University Press, 1983; 9.58–9.70.

500 people are affected, but in some populations, such as the Lebanese
and South Africans of Afrikaans descent, the incidence is much higher.

FH is a very serious disorder, with a much greater risk of development of premature CHD than common hyperlipidaemia: a fact which is
partly due to elevated LDL from birth. About 1 in 20 patients presenting with a myocardial infarction under the age of 60 have this condition. Slack originally reported in the 1960s that, untreated, up to 85
per cent of men with FH will have a myocardial infarction and 50 per
cent will have died by the age of 60 years. More recent data on risk

Table 7.2 Mortality analysis: coronary heart disease (ICD (ninth revision) codes 410–14) (from BMJ (1991), 303, 893–6, with permission)

Age (years)	Person years of observation	Observed deaths	Expected deaths	Standardized[4] mortality ratio	95% confidence interval
Men					
20–39	439	5	0.06	8 975[2]	2710 to 19 400
40–59	653	4	1.28	312	85 to 800
60–74	133	1	1.34	75	2 to 416
20–74	1226	10	2.67	374[3]	180 to 689
Women					
20–39	335	1	0.01	16 039[1]	253 to 55 700
40–59	447	4	0.26	1 538	419 to 3940
60–74	225	0	0.94		
20–74	1008	5	1.21	413[1]	134 to 964
Men and Women					
20–39	774	6	0.06	9 686[3]	3670 to 21 800
40–59	1110	8	1.54	519[3]	224 to 1020
60–74	358	1	2.28	44	1 to 244
20–74	2234	15	3.88	386[3]	210 to 639

[1] $p < 0.05$; [2] $p < 0.01$; [3] $p < 0.01$
[4] standardized mortality ratio—mortality rate in FH patients compared to that of UK population rate in that age group (100 = same rate as general population)

from the Simon Broome register in the UK are shown in Table 7.2. It is of note that these are patients who have had their condition detected and some treatment—even though this may not have been initiated early enough. A worse prognosis would be expected for those who have not had any attention. Patients may be disabled by CHD in their thirties. The family history below illustrates the devastating effects it can have (Fig. 7.1). A study of 700 patients with FH indicates that coronary narrowing may be detected at an average age of 17 years in men and 25 years in women.

Women with FH seem to have a better prognosis than men, with CHD developing some 10–15 years later, but the relative risk for a young women with FH is very high.

FH is characterized by xanthomas in the extensor tendons of the hands, the Achilles tendons (Figs. 7.2 and 7.3), and, occasionally, at the insertion of the patella tendon. Corneal arcus commonly occurs in FH, though it may occur in other types of hypercholesterolaemia and is

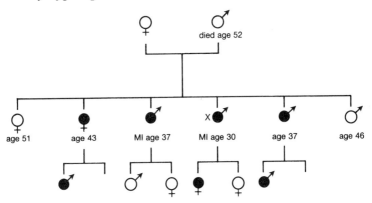

● =individual with familial hypercholesterolaemia

Affected adults all had tendon xanthomas and a plasma cholesterol>9 mmol/l at diagnosis. The family was screened after patient X had a myocardial infection at age 30 and was found to have a cholesterol of 13 mmol/l. Screening has allowed diagnosis in six other family members and commencement of cholesterol-lowering therapy.

Fig. 7.1 Family tree showing individuals with familial hypercholesterolaemia.

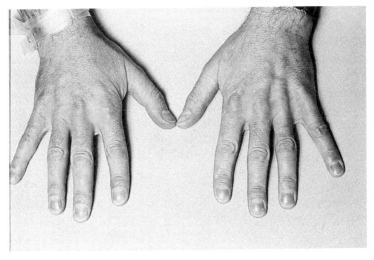

Fig. 7.2 Xanthomas in extensor tendons.

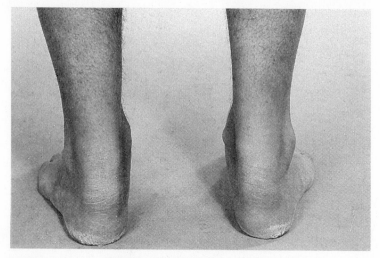

Fig. 7.3 Achilles tendon xanthomas.

frequently seen in old people with normal lipids. Half arcus in a young person is, however, very suggestive of FH (Fig. 7.4). Xanthelasma (Fig. 7.5) are less specific clinical signs, because they may be found in people with a normal cholesterol and in those with common hyperlipidaemia.

Total cholesterol levels in heterozygous patients may range from 7 to 15 mmol/l, but are commonly between 8.5 and 12 mmol/l in affected adults. Levels in affected children are usually somewhat lower. Lp(a) levels are sometimes high, and the concentration of Lp(a) appears a strong predictor of CHD risk in these patients.

Triglyceride and VLDL levels are normal or slightly raised and HDL cholesterol is usually decreased. The presence of xanthomas and elevated levels of total plasma cholesterol (chiefly found in LDL) are sufficient evidence to make the diagnosis. The xanthomas may, however, be slight and must be carefully sought. If xanthomas are absent, as they often are in childhood or early adult life, the condition may be diagnosed if LDL cholesterol is greater than 5 mmol/l and FH has been diagnosed in a first-degree relative. It is usually possible to diagnose this condition in children, although LDL should be measured in most cases because both the total and the LDL cholesterol are lower

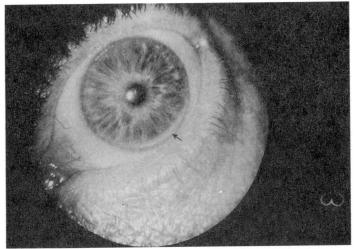

Fig. 7.4 Corneal arcus in a 35-year-old.

in children (see Chapter 5). Neonatal diagnosis can be made from cord blood, but it is more common for the results to be inconclusive when measures are made at this time and a repeat test is usually performed later. Genetic counselling is discussed in Chapter 10.

Energetic treatment is essential for people with FH. Dietary modification is considered in Chapter 8, and this may result in a modest

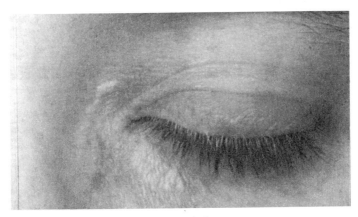

Fig. 7.5 Xanthelasma.

reduction of cholesterol levels, particularly if the patient was obese. However, diet alone seldom achieves satisfactory lipid levels and lipid-lowering drugs are necessary. Bile acid sequestrants and HMG coA reductase inhibitors are often used, but fibric acid derivatives are possible additional or alternative drugs. In some centres ileal bypass surgery has been performed in resistant cases, but this procedure has frequently resulted in severe gastrointestinal side-effects and is now very seldom performed. All these cholesterol-lowering treatments are associated with a reduction in size of xanthomas. Clinical trials including patients with FH indicate benefit in terms of morbidity and mortality from CHD.

In the rare homozygous form of FH the patients have virtually no LDL receptors on their cells and the plasma cholesterol levels are often greater than 20 mmol/l. Thus xanthomas, aortic stenosis, and CHD may occur in childhood. Drug treatment seldom achieves normal lipid levels, and LDL apheresis together with combined drug treatment appears to be the therapy of choice. Even with treatment, the prognosis is poor and few survive beyond the age of 20.

Possible familial hypercholesterolaemia

Primary hypercholesterolaemia may be found in several family members although none have tendon xanthomas. Without performing receptor studies, which is impractical, it is not possible to tell whether each family has a receptor defect or whether there is a different inherited metabolic defect. In some families it is difficult to elicit a family history suggestive of an inherited hyperlipidaemia. This is particularly the case if a disorder is passed from the women in a family as death from another disease, such as cancer, may occur before the women develop clinical CHD.

Table 7.3 shows the FH register criteria for the diagnosis of FH and possible FH. The category of 'possible FH' is unfortunately likely to include a number of cases of familial combined hyperlipidaemia.

Familial combined hyperlipidaemia

This inherited disorder was only recognized as a separate condition in the 1970s and it is still incompletely understood. It does, however, appear to be common with an incidence as high as 1 in 300. The precise

Table 7.2 Criteria for diagnosis of familial hypercholesterolaemia (FH) used for the Familial Hyperlipidaemia Register—a British register of patients with this condition

Definite FH		
Cholesterol	> 7.5 mmol/l (adult)	
	>6.5 mmol/l (child under 16)	
or		
LDL cholesterol	> 4.9 mmol/l (adult)	
Plus		
Tendon xanthomas in patient or relative		
Possible FH		Family history myocardial infarction
Cholesterol	>7.5 mmol/l (adult)	under 50 (second degree relative)
	>6.5 mmol/l (child under 16)	under 60 (first degree relative)
	Plus	or
		Family history raised
or		cholesterol in first degree relative
LDL cholesterol	4.9 mmol/l (adult)	

mode of inheritance has not been resolved, but it is probably autosomal dominant. It is characterized by elevated levels of VLDL and often of LDL (and as a result, both cholesterol and triglyceride) and low levels of HDL. The high VLDL is generally due to increased synthesis; and apo B levels are generally high due to increased hepatic synthesis. Cholesterol levels are usually 8–10 mmol/l and triglycerides 3–6 mmol/l. This condition should be suspected in families with a strong history of premature CHD and the characteristic metabolic disturbance in several family members, but no xanthomas. The expression of the metabolic abnormality may differ in members of the same family, probably as a result of interaction between genetic and environmental factors, especially diet. Some family members may have predominant hypertriglyceridaemia, some hypercholesterolaemia, and the pattern may also vary with age. Unlike FH, the disorder is not present until adult life and in small families the distinction between this condition and 'common' hyperlipidaemia may be difficult and sometimes impossible. It is nevertheless important to attempt to establish the diagnosis since the prognosis of familial combined hyperlipidaemia is much worse than that of common hyperlipidaemia. The hyperlipidaemia may sometimes respond to dietary modification alone, but if it does not the fibrate drugs may be used, sometimes in combination with a bile acid sequestrant.

Remnant hyperlipoproteinaemia

In this condition elevated levels of cholesterol (around 10–15 mmol/l) and triglyceride (5–12 mmol/l) are due to accumulation of IDL and the denser sub-classes of VLDL, as well as some chylomicrons. LDL and HDL levels are low. VLDL in this condition has a number of atypical features: slow electrophoretic mobility (giving a broad B band), a high ratio of cholesterol to triglyceride (a molar ratio greater than 1:1 in the VLDL fraction), and a high content of apo E. Although lipoprotein electrophoresis is now rarely performed, this condition is still sometimes called broad beta disease, or type III hyperlipidaemia. The disorder appears to be due to impaired lipoprotein catabolism which results in an accumulation of remnant particles.

The genetics of this condition are complex. Most affected individuals have an apo E2E2 genotype and do not produce apo E3, but as this phenotype is present in 1 per cent of a healthy population, other factors must be involved. It has been suggested that apo-E3 deficiency may interact with other inherited hyperlipidaemias (e.g. FH, familial combined), hypothyroidism, or diabetes to produce remnant hyperlipidaemia. While the genetics and mechanism may be complicated, the clinical manifestations are clearly defined. Many patients have the typical cutaneous lesions; linear, orange coloured, planar xanthomas seen in the palmer creases and/or tubo-eruptive xanthomas, which are commonly found on the elbows and which are diagnostic (Fig. 7.6).

Although the precise risks have not been quantified there is no doubt about the increased vascular risk. Peripheral vascular disease, cerebrovascular disease, and CHD commonly occur. The diagnosis is usually suspected because of the skin lesions and confirmed by finding combined hyperlipidaemia (a similar elevation of cholesterol and triglyceride) and a broad beta band on lipoprotein electrophoresis. Occasionally further tests such as apo-E typing and confirmation of a VLDL cholesterol:triglyceride molar ratio >1 may be needed. The xanthomas and metabolic abnormality may respond promptly to the treatment of any secondary factors, but if not then they usually respond rapidly to diet and a fibrate.

Familial hypertriglyceridaemia

There are several inherited forms of hypertriglyceridaemia. If the triglyceride levels are very high, say over 20 mmol/l, then there may be the classical clinical features of eruptive xanthomas (Fig. 7.7), lipaemia retinalis, abdominal pain, hepatosplenomegaly, and an increased risk of acute pancreatitis. Lipid exudates may occur in the retina from vessel leakage and impair vision if they are close to the macula. Hypertriglyceridaemia may also be associated with retinal vessel occlusion. The association with CHD is less clear and may depend on other factors such as HDL cholesterol; it is more significant if the HDL cholesterol is low.

Endogenous hypertriglyceridaemia

The main abnormality is an increase in VLDL probably due to excessive synthesis. There may also be chylomicronaemia which disappears with a fat-free diet while the VLDL abnormality persists. Triglycerides range from 5 to 50 mmol/l. Cholesterol is only modestly increased and

LDL and HDL levels are low. Affected relatives show a consistent metabolic abnormality, and impaired glucose tolerance, or diabetes and obesity, are often associated. The interrelationships are not clearly

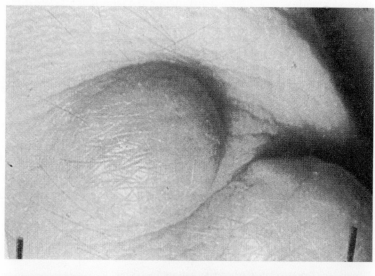

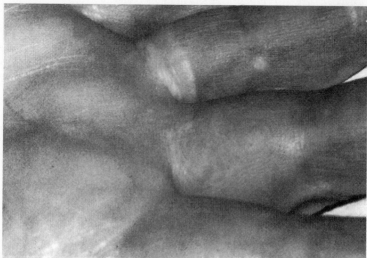

Fig. 7.6 (a) Tubo-eruptive xanthomas and (b) palmar crease xanthomas. (Courtesy of Professor B. Lewis.)

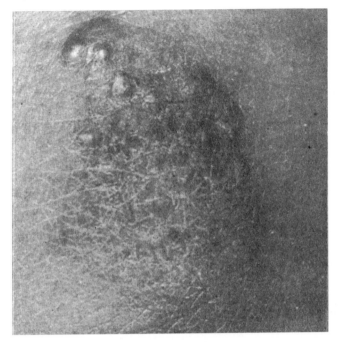

Fig. 7.7 Eruptive xanthomas.

understood, but hyperinsulinaemia may be relevant. Plasma stored overnight in the refrigerator shows diffuse opalescence, with or without a creamy upper layer of chylomicrons. Dietary modification may be relatively ineffective, but should be advised, together with weight reduction and reduction in alcohol intake. Gemfibrozil, bezafibrate, nicotinic acid, progestogens, and omega-3 preparations have been used with varying success.

Lipoprotein-lipase or apo-CII deficiency

A deficiency of lipoprotein lipase or its activator apo CII are very uncommon conditions which lead to severe hypertriglyceridaemia characterized by an inability to clear ingested fat. The inheritance is autosomal recessive and a common history in affected individuals is of recurrent episodes of abdominal pain or pancreatitis and/or eruptive xanthomas. Stored plasma shows a creamy upper layer of chylomicrons. LDL and HDL levels are low. Plasma triglycerides may be elevated from birth and may be as high as 20–100 mmol/l. Lipoprotein lipase deficiency is identified by specific assay available in one or two specialized laboratories. Apo CII can be measured, but a deficiency can be indicated simply by demonstrating a substantial reduction in the hypertriglyceridaemia after the infusion of fresh frozen plasma, which provides the apoproteins. Virtual removal of fat from the diet for three days in hospital results in a marked fall in triglyceride levels and the chylomicrons often disappear. Long-term treatment involves severe restriction of all fat-rich foods. Medium chain triglycerides may be used.

These conditions are very rare: accumulation of chylomicrons (the 'chylomicronaemia syndrome') is more commonly seen as a secondary phenomenon.

Common 'polygenic' hyperlipidaemia

A considerable number of people with hyperlipidaemia of moderate severity, despite sensible diet, do not have a family history of hypercholesterolaemia or premature CHD. The cause in these individuals may be multifactorial and involve genetic and environmental factors which have not yet been elucidated. At present it is a diagnosis made after the exclusion of other causes. People with common hypercholesterolaemia do not have xanthomas. The first line of treatment is a lipid-lowering diet. The need for any drug treatment will depend on the patient's age, condition, and lipid levels. More active treatment is usually considered if the individual has other risk factors for CHD.

Familial lipoprotein deficiency

These disorders result not in high but in low lipoprotein levels.

The inherited lipoprotein deficiency disorders are of two major types—those affecting lipoproteins containing apolipoprotein B (chylomicrons, VLDL, and LDL), and those affecting lipoproteins containing the A apolipoproteins (HDL). The disorders may result in either low or unmeasurable concentrations of the apoproteins and the particular lipoprotein particles. Low levels of apo A and HDL are increasingly being recognized in some families with premature CHD. More work is needed on these conditions, but such a problem should be considered in

Table 7.4 Hypolipoproteinaemias

Type	Onset (Inheritance)	Lipids	Clinical effects
Abeta	Early childhood (autosomal recessive)	Cholesterol 1–2 mmol/l Tg < 0.2 mmol/l No apo B	Fat malabsorption, ataxia, neuropathy, retinitis pigmentosa
Hypo-beta	Childhood/adult (autosomal dominant)	Cholesterol 1–3 mmol/l Low apo B	Some degree of fat malabsorption
Tangier's	Childhood (autosomal recessive)	Cholesterol 1–3 mmol/l Tg normal HDL cholesterol very low	Large orange tonsils, corneal opacities, polyneuropathy. ? increased CHD risk
Hypo-alpha	Child to adult	HDL cholesterol low Apo A low	Increased CHD risk

families with a strong history of CHD and none of the more commonly recognized risk factors.

Other lipoprotein deficiency states—such as Tangier's disease and hypo- and abeta-hypolipoproteinaemia—are rare. The clinical features of the three major types are summarized in Table 7.4.

The disorders in which the apo-B concentration is low are usually associated with a low incidence of CHD. However some disorders where there is also a low apo A and a very reduced HDL cholesterol may be associated with an increased risk of CHD, even if the LDL cholesterol is relatively low. This is the case in Tangier's disease. This condition is rare, but there is a notable finding of markedly enlarged, orange tonsils which may cause respiratory obstruction.

8

Dietary management of hyperlipidaemia

In recent years there have been several important reports concerning diet and cardiovascular disease. These are mainly concerned with general advice for the population—the healthy eating plan—and are discussed in Chapter 11. Stricter dietary control than that recommended for the general population is often required for people with diagnosed hyperlipidaemia. This can be introduced in two stages. The reduction in energy from fat to 30 per cent or less of total energy can be considered as stage A. Some people will be deemed to need the addition of drug therapy while continuing on the stage A diet. Some people may need, and accept, a further reduction which can be considered as stage B.

The main dietary principles

There are several complementary dietary changes which help to reduce cholesterol. Attention to all of them will achieve the greatest cholesterol reduction, but the emphasis needs to be varied, taking into account the patient's preferences and needs.

The main aspects are :

1. Attainment of ideal body weight.
2. Reduction of saturated fatty acids, partially compensated for by an increase in poly- and monounsaturated fatty acids.
3. Increase in fibre-rich carbohydrate.
4. Substantial reduction in alcohol intake in overweight patients or those with hypertriglyceridaemia.

Modification of dietary protein source and cholesterol intake may also be helpful. In addition, an increase in fruit and vegetables is advised to increase the intake of vitamin C, β-carotene, lycopene, and other potential antioxidants.

Attainment of ideal body weight

Obesity is a major cause of hypertriglyceridaemia and weight loss can often produce an appreciable reduction in triglyceride levels. Cholesterol levels may also be reduced to some extent by weight reduction and HDL-cholesterol tends to rise. The aim should be to achieve a body mass index (weight/height^2) of 20–25. Table 8.1 shows the approximate weight range which corresponds to this in men and women of different height. For people who are substantially overweight it is important to set intermediate goals since people often become disheartened if they feel that they have an impossible target. A weight loss of 2 kg per month should be regarded as perfectly satisfactory and 4 kg per month as excellent. Even those who are moderately overweight are likely to achieve improvement in their blood lipids as a result of modest weight loss. Many patients do not need to count calories—changing from inappropriate to appropriate foods often achieves a satisfactory weight reduction. When this is not achieved it is essential for the dietitian (or other appropriately qualified person) to assess approximate energy intake and to advise as to how this might be reduced by about one third.

Recommendations of fixed energy diets (e.g. 1000 kcal or 4200 mJ reducing diets) can be inappropriate and disheartening, especially for those whose present energy intake is very high.

Reduction of saturated fatty acids and increase in mono-unsaturated and polyunsaturated fatty acids

Although fat intake has fallen in several countries with high CHD rates many people have between 35 and 40 per cent of their total energy as fat. The reduction in total fat to no more than 30 per cent total energy required for stage A is achieved by a reduction in saturated fatty acids (SAFA) to no more than 10 per cent total energy. The actual amount of fat allowed will thus depend on the required energy intake of the person, e.g. for someone requiring 1000 kcal/day (4200 kJ), this would be 35 g fat of which <11 g would be SAFA, and for someone requiring 2500 kcal/day (10500 kJ), this would be 85 g fat of which <25 g would be SAFA. SAFA may be partially replaced by mono- and polyunsaturated fatty acids (MUFA, PUFA). Both MUFA and PUFA have been shown to help reduce TC and LDL-C but the recommendation to increase their intake needs to be tempered with several caveats. First,

Table 8.1 Guidelines for body weight (based on Bray (1979), Metropolitan Life Insurance Tables (1960) and Report on Obesity, Royal College of Physicians, London (1984)). The minimum level for diagnosing obesity is taken as 20 per cent above the upper limit of the acceptable weight range

Height without shoes		Weight without clothes (kg)		
Ft. ins.	Metres	Acceptable average	Acceptable range	Obese
Men				
5′ 3″	1.60	58	52–65	78
5′ 4″	1.63	59	54–67	80
5′ 5″	1.65	60	55–69	82
5′ 6″	1.68	62	56–71	85
5′ 7″	1.70	64	58–73	88
5′ 8″	1.73	66	59–74	89
5′ 9″	1.75	67	61–76	91
5′ 10″	1.78	69	65–80	96
6′ 0″	1.83	73	66–83	100
6′ 1″	1.85	75	69–86	103
6′ 2″	1.88	77	71–88	106
Body mass index		22	20.1–25	30
Women				
5′ 0″	1.52	48	44–57	68
5′ 1″	1.55	50	45–58	70
5′ 2″	1.57	51	46–59	71
5′ 3″	1.60	53	48–61	73
5′ 4″	1.63	55	49–63	76
5′ 5″	1.65	56	51–65	78
5′ 6″	1.68	58	52–66	79
5′ 7″	1.70	60	53–67	80
5′ 8″	1.73	62	55–69	83
5′ 9″	1.75	63	57–71	85
5′ 10″	1.78	65	58–73	88
Body mass index		20.8	18.7–23.8	28.6

Conversion: 8 stone = 50 kg; 9 stone = 57 kg; 10 stone = 64 kg; 11 stone = 70 kg

all types of fats are equally high in calories (9 kcal/g compared with 4 kcal/g for carbohydrate and protein) and when weight reduction is important it is necessary for total fat to be reduced. Second, while

MUFA appears to be a particularly good replacement fat for SAFA because of beneficial effects on HDL (and a probable ability to reduce oxidation of lipoproteins) it is important to be aware that these benefits are only associated with the naturally occurring *cis* forms of MUFA and not with *trans* forms produced in the manufacturing process. Large quantities of *trans* fatty acids may increase LDL and reduce HDL. Thus, the most appropriate MUFA sources are olive oil and canola and products prepared from them which are low in *trans* forms. Finally, it is important to appreciate that there are two types of naturally occurring PUFA: n-6 PUFA which are derived from plant sources (such as corn oil and sunflower seed oil) and n-3 PUFA derived from some nuts, avocados, and oily fish. n-6 PUFA help to lower LDL-C but in large amounts may have an unfavourable effect by also reducing HDL. The very long chain polyunsaturated fatty acids from fish help to lower VLDL and may reduce the tendency towards thrombosis. They have a variable effect on LDL, and while an increase in fish consumption is recommended, especially as a partial replacement for meat, the widespread use of expensive refined supplements is definitely not (see Chapter 9). Further examples of how foods high in SAFA may be replaced by low-fat foods or foods relatively high in MUFA and PUFA are shown in Table 8.2. Simple dietary changes along these lines, particularly if accompanied by weight loss when necessary, can often produce an appreciable improvement in the lipid profile. If a further reduction of SAFA is required in order to achieve an intake which is less than 8 per cent total energy (stage B) the assistance of a dietitian is essential.

In people with an inability to clear ingested fat (those with lipoprotein lipase or apo CII deficiency) it is necessary to reduce fat to an extremely low level of intake to 10–20 g/day.

Such diets usually need supplementation with medium-chain triglycerides (MCT) and vitamins and are usually only recommended by dietitians in specialist clinics.

Increase in fibre-rich carbohydrate

Carbohydrate may be increased to compensate for the reduction in fat and it is appropriate that most of the carbohydrate should be unprocessed and rich in dietary fibre. While insoluble fibre (bran and other fibre from cereal sources) may be of general benefit and helpful in reducing some forms of gastrointestinal disease, it is only the soluble

Table 8.2 Example of ways in which high-fat products may be exchanged for low fat alternatives or products which are higher in MUFA or PUFA

Product	Fat (g/100 g)		Alternative	Fat (g/100 g)	
	Total	PUFA		Total	PUFA
Whole milk	3.8	0.1	Skimmed milk	0.1–0.5	–
			Semi-skimmed milk	1.5	0.2
Salad cream			Low-calorie salad cream	13	
Double cream	48	1	Yoghurt	1	–
Cream cheese	47	1	Cottage cheese	4	
Cheddar cheese	38	1	Edam/camembert	23	1
Stilton	40		'Low-fat' cheeses	15–25	1
Butter	82	2	'High PUFA' margarine	81	50–60
Hard margarine	81	14	Low-fat spread	41	12
Lard	99	9	Sunflower oil	100	52
Coconut oil	90	2	Soya oil	100	57
Grilled streaky bacon	36	3	Roast chicken	5.5	1
Grilled beefburger	20	1	Rabbit—stewed	8	3
Sausages (pork)	25	2	Lean ham	5	1
Pork chop—grilled	24	2	Kidney	5	1
Luncheon meat	27	2	Tuna fish (in vegetable oil)	22	8
Pork pie	27	2	Grilled white fish	1.5	0.5

Note All figures are an approximate value (based on tables of McCance and Widdowson in *The composition of foods* (4th edn) HMSO).
These figures should be used to compare the percentage fat of a weight of similar products when considering substitution. They do *not* provide a guide to the percentage of energy from that food which will be from fat or saturated fat.

or gel-forming fibres (such as those in various cooked dried beans and in oats) and pectins (in fruit) which have been shown to have some effect in lowering LDL levels. The effects of soluble fibre are relatively small by comparison with the effects of manipulating dietary fat and some effect may actually be the result of high-fibre foods replacing higher-fat foods.

It is usually appropriate to recommend a decrease in 'extrinsic' sugars (all sugars which are not an integral part of the cellular structure of foods) except for milk sugar (lactose). Examples of these sugars are sucrose or table sugar (whether white or brown), sugars in jam, honey, and baked or confectionery products. They are rich in energy but have few essential nutrients. Furthermore they may have some effect in raising triglycerides, and possibly also blood glucose in some people, so restriction is particularly appropriate in those who are obese, hyper-triglyceridaemic, or glucose intolerant. 'Intrinsic' sugars (those which are incorporated in the cellular structure of foods) are not restricted. These occur within fruits and vegetables. Such foods may be particularly beneficial as they are also high in vitamin C and carotenes which are dietary antioxidants that may reduce the risk of athero-sclerosis by reducing oxidation of lipoproteins.

Alcohol

There is epidemiological evidence that for most of the population a modest alcohol intake may be beneficial or neutral. It may increase HDL, and substances in wine may have antioxidant properties. Some people are, however, particularly sensitive to its effects on plasma lipids, body weight, and blood pressure. Moderate quantities of alcohol tend to increase triglyceride levels. Alcohol must therefore be severely restricted or preferably eliminated by people with hypertriglycerid-aemia and those who are overweight. People with other disorders should probably restrict their intake to about 12 units per week.

Protein

Vegetable proteins derived from legumes (such as soya) may help to lower LDL cholesterol.

Salt

In view of the fact that dietary sodium can influence blood pressure it is appropriate to advise sodium restriction to patients following a lipid-lowering diet. An intake of less than 90 mmol sodium per day would seem sensible. This is in keeping with the general recommendations for healthier eating, and the first step involves avoiding adding salt at the table and using as little as possible in cooking. Many manufactured products are high in sodium so wherever possible they should be restricted or low sodium alternatives should be selected.

Dietary cholesterol

Dietary cholesterol (from eggs, shellfish, and diary products) increases blood cholesterol when taken in large quantities by people who have a relatively high intake of saturated fat. Reducing fat intake will in itself reduce dietary cholesterol. On a diet reduced in fat, intake is usually well below 300 mg per day and there is no evidence that restricting dietary cholesterol further gives much additional benefit.

Table 8.3 summarizes the optimal nutrient composition of a lipid-lowering diet.

Practical dietary advice

If people are to be encouraged to change their diet they need to be aware of the potential benefits. They also need sufficient knowledge about the composition of various foods to make the appropriate changes.

For those who have been on an average 'Western' diet, their saturated fat intake will generally have come from four main sources. Meat and meat products will have supplied about a quarter of the total, and butter and margarine another quarter. Milk often accounts for an eighth, and milk and cheese together constitute a third for some people. Cooking fats often account for another third. Chocolate, pastries, biscuits, cakes, and convenience foods are often high in saturated fat, but because it is 'hidden' it is often ignored when an individual considers his or her fat intake. Many packaged and processed foods give insufficient information about the food composition of the contents although this situation is slowly improving. Hard margarines may be labelled as vegetable fats but the hydrogenating process will have converted much of the PUFA to saturated or *trans* fatty acids. Values for percentage fat expressed as grams of fat per 100 g food weight are often uninformative as the amount of water present is so different between, for example, milk and sausages. Values which are most helpful in diet planning are the percentage of

Table 8.3 Summary of the optimal nutrient composition of a lipid-lowering diet. *Total energy* should be tailored to individual requirements. Weight loss in the obese helps to normalize lipid levels in most conditions

Nutrient		
Fat	< 30%	*Stage A*: SAFA should provide about 10% total energy, the rest should be from *cis* MUFA or PUFA, so that the *ratio of* P:M:S should be 1:1:1. *Stage B*: SAFA should be about 8%; some replacement with MUFA or PUFA as above is appropriate but total fat intake should remain below 28% total energy. In lipoprotein lipase or apo CII deficiency more severe restriction required.
Carbohydrate	50–60%	Unprocessed fibre-rich carbohydrate should predominate Ideally 20 g fibre/1000 kCal. Wide range of fresh vegetables and fruit strongly recommended. Pectins and other gel-forming fibres (e.g. those derived from various cooked beans) are useful for LDL lowering.
Protein	10–15%	Vegetable proteins derived from legumes (e.g. soya) may help to decrease LDL.
Extrinsic sugars		Should be severely restricted in the obese or if triglycerides are raised.
Alcohol		Should be severely restricted in the obese or if triglycerides are raised. A sensible maximum for others is 12 units per week.
Cholesterol		Less than 300 mg/day.

Table 8.4 Fat content of different foods by percentage of total energy

Product	Serving	kCals	Protein	Fat	Carbohydrate
			% total energy available from:		
Skimmed milk	$^1/_3$ pt	66	40	1	59
Whole milk	$^1/_3$ pt	130	20	52	28
Yoghurt (low-fat, flavoured)	small carton	122	23	10	67
Cream (double)	2 tbsp	179	1	97	2
Cottage cheese	100 g	96	56	38	6
Cheddar cheese	60 g	244	26	74	—
Roast chicken	120 g	178	68	32	—
Grilled white fish	100 g	95	88	12	—
Lean ham	2 thin slices	72	61	39	—
Pork sausages	2 grilled	382	16	70	14
Pork chop	250 g	645	34	66	—
Pork pie	mini	451	10	64	26
Beefburger	small	158	31	59	10
Chips	60 g portion	152	6	37	57
Boiled potatoes	2	96	6	–	94
Chocolate (milk)	small bar	265	6	50	44
Biscuits	1 digestive	71	8	38	54
Fruit cake	1 med. slice	212	5	31	64
Crisps	small packet	133	4	60	36
Bread (wholemeal)	1 med. slice	108	15	9	76
Rice (boiled)	180 g	222	5	2	94
Cornflakes	medium bowl	111	9	3	90
Apples	1	55	2	—	98
Vegetables (green)	100 g	18	30	—	70
Baked beans	small tin	144	31	7	62

total energy of the food provided by fat, and these are given in Table 8.4. Some foods such as pork pies may be a quarter fat by weight and three quarters of the energy may be from fat.

In addition to a high fat intake, most people will have been consuming relatively little dietary fibre, and practical advice on the ways to increase their intake is needed.

For many people the provision of a simple diet sheet together with recipes and advice on food preparation will be a major step in the right direction. Nothing can replace individual consultation with a dietitian, but where this is not available the advice sheet shown in Table 8.5, the principles outlined in Table 8.6, and the hints and sample recipes given in the Appendix should be helpful. Many people have rather conservative ideas about food and need advice and ideas to create interesting low-fat meals. They should be encouraged to try foods which may not have been part of their previous diet, such as kidney beans, chick peas, lentils, and wholemeal pasta, and so on. Several food manufacturers now produce low-fat products including skimmed milk, yoghurts, soft and hard cheeses, and prepared meals. These do contain less fat than their counterparts, but even the 'low-fat' hard cheeses often contain a substantial quantity of fat, and intake must remain controlled. This also applies to some low-fat spreads which are lower in calories, but still contain a considerable proportion of saturated fat. Some idea of the fat content of an average helping of a number of foods, and the percentage energy from fat, protein and carbohydrate are given in Table 8.4.

Foods in the advisable column in Tables 8.5 and 8.6 are generally low in fat or high in fibre and should be used regularly. Foods 'not advised' contain large proportions of saturated fats and therefore should be avoided wherever possible. Foods 'in moderation' contain smaller amounts of fat or polyunsaturated fats or are high in 'empty' calories. Advice about the consumption of foods in these columns depends on the stage of the diet recommended and consideration of other factors, such as the person's need to lose weight (or not). The interpretation of moderation obviously varies and more details are usually needed: for example, in a stage A diet, medium-fat cheese is usually restricted to twice a week. In a stage B diet, intake will probably have to be limited to once a week only. Stage B diets are thus stringent, but are acceptable to some people who are well motivated or very keen to avoid drug treatment.

A step-wise programme for dietary modification in a healthy young adult is given in Fig. 8.1. The diet recommendations suggested would need to be initiated at lower lipid levels in those with CHD or other risk factors.

Most patients eating a traditional Western diet, who comply rigidly with a lipid-lowering diet, will achieve a reduction of approximately 20 per cent in their plasma cholesterol. This may be greater if weight loss is also achieved where appropriate. However there is a great deal of individual variation in response, and the precise diagnosis is also an important factor in determining response. Patients with familial hypercholesterolaemia usually respond less to diet than those with common

Table 8.5 Stage A diet

	Eat regularly	Eat in moderation	Treats	Avoid eating
Cereals	Wholemeal flour, oatmeal wholemeal bread, wholegrain cereals, porridge oats, crispbreads, brown rice, wholemeal pasta, cornmeal, untoasted sugar-free muesli	White bread White flour White rice and pasta Water biscuits	Sugar-coated cereals Plain semi-sweet biscuits Ordinary muesli	Sweet biscuits, cream-filled biscuits, cream crackers, cheese biscuits, croissants
Fruit and vegetables	All fresh, frozen, dried, and unsweetened tinned fruit All fresh, frozen, dried, and tinned vegetables, (especially peas, baked beans, broad beans, and lentils) Baked potatoes (eat skins) Walnuts Chestnuts		Fruit in syrup Crystallized fruit Avocado Chips and roast potatoes cooked in suitable oil Peanuts and most other nuts e.g. almonds, hazelnuts, brazil nuts	Chips and roast potatoes Crisps and savoury snacks Coconut
Meat and fish	All fresh and frozen fish, e.g. cod, plaice, herring, mackerel Tinned fish in brine and tomato sauce e.g. sardines and tuna Chicken, turkey, veal, rabbit Game Soya protein meat substitute	Fish fried in suitable oil or tinned in oil (drained) Lean beef, pork, lamb, ham and gammon. Very lean minced meat	Prawns, lobster, crab, oysters, molluscs, winkles Liver, kidney, tripe, sweetbreads Grilled back bacon	Fried scampi Sausages, luncheon meats, corned beef, pate, salami, streaky bacon. Duck, goose, meat pies and pasties, Scotch eggs Visible fat on meats, crackling, chicken skin

Table 8.5 cont'd.

	Eat regularly	Eat in moderation	Treats	Avoid eating
Dairy produce	Skimmed milk, soya milk, powdered skimmed milk Cottage cheese Low-fat curd cheese Low-fat yoghurt	Semi-skimmed milk	Medium-fat cheeses, e.g. Edam, Camembert, Gouda, Brie, cheese spreads	Whole milk and cream Full-fat yoghurt Cheese e.g. Stilton, Cheddar, cream cheese Evaporated or condensed milk
	Egg white		Half-fat cheeses	
			labelled 'low fat' Sweetened condensed skim milk	Imitation cream Excess eggs
	Small amounts from next column	Soft margarine labelled 'high in polyunsaturates' Corn oil, sunflower oil, soya oil, safflower oil, rapeseed oil, olive oil		All hard margarines, shortenings, and oils not labelled 'high in monounsaturates and/or polyunsaturates' Butter, lard, suet, and dripping Vegetable oil or margarine of unknown origin
Other foods	Jelly (low sugar) Sorbet Fat-free homemade soups Low-fat, low-sugar yoghurt Low-fat natural yoghurt	Pastry, puddings, cakes, biscuits, sauces, etc. made with wholemeal flour and fat or oil as above	Packet soups	Pastries, puddings, cakes, and sauces made with whole milk and fat or oil as above Suet dumpling or puddings Ice cream Cream soups

Table 8.5 cont'd.

Eat regularly	Eat in moderation	Treats	Avoid eating
Marmite, Bovril, chutneys, and pickles Sugar-free artificial sweeteners	Fish and meat pastes Peanut butter Low-sugar jams and marmalade.	Boiled sweets, fruit pastilles, and jellies. Jam, marmalade, honey	Chocolate spreads Chocolate, toffees, fudge butterscotch Carob chocolate Coconut bars
Tea, coffee, mineral water, fruit juices (unsweetened)	Alcohol	Sweetened drinks Squashes, fruit juice Malted milk or hot chocolate drinks made with skimmed milk	Whole milk drinks Cream-based liqueurs
Herbs, spices, Tabasco, Worcestershire sauce, soy sauce, lemon juice	Homemade dressings and low-fat mayonnaise made with suitable oils	Parmesan cheese	Ordinary or cream dressings and mayonnaises

Eat regularly—Choose from this group daily.
Eat in moderation—Moderate amounts 2–3 times per week.
treat—Moderate amounts once a week or less.

Table 8.6 Stricter diet for persistent hyperlipidaemia—stage B

	Eat regularly	Eat in moderation	Avoid eating	
Cereals	Wholemeal flour, oatmeal wholemeal bread, wholegrain cereals, porridge oats, crispbreads, brown rice, wholemeal pasta, cornmeal, untoasted sugar-free muesli	White bread White flour White rice and pasta (If wholemeal varieties unavailable)	Sugar-coated cereals Plain semi-sweet biscuits Ordinary muesli	Sweet biscuits, cream-filled biscuits, cream crackers, cheese biscuits, croissants
Fruit and vegetables	All fresh, frozen, dried, and unsweetened tinned fruit All fresh, frozen, dried, and tinned vegetables, (especially peas, baked beans, broad beans, and lentils) Baked potatoes (eat skins) Walnuts Chestnuts		Fruit in syrup Crystallized fruit Avocado Chips and roast potatoes cooked in suitable oil Peanuts and most other nuts e.g. almonds, hazelnuts, brazilnuts (N.B. some allowed if vegetarian)	Chips and roast potatoes Crisps and savoury snacks Coconut
Meat and fish	All fresh and frozen fish, e.g. cod, plaice, herring, mackerel Tinned fish in brine and tomato sauce e.g. sardines and tuna Chicken, turkey, veal, rabbit Game Soya protein meat substitute	Fish fried in suitable oil (once a week) Lean beef, pork, lamb, ham and gammon. Very lean minced meat	Prawns, lobster, crab, oysters, molluscs, winkles Liver, kidney, tripe, sweetbreads Grilled back bacon	Fried scampi Sausages, luncheon meats, corned beef, pate, salami, streaky bacon. Duck, goose, meat pies and pasties, Scotch eggs Visible fat on meats, crackling, chicken skin

Table 8.6 cont'd.

	Eat regularly	Eat in moderation	Avoid eating
Dairy produce	Skimmed milk, soya milk, powdered skimmed milk Cottage cheese Low-fat curd cheese Low-fat yoghurt Egg white	Low-fat cheese spread	Medium-fat cheeses, e.g. Edam, Camembert, Gouda, Brie, cheese spreads	Whole milk and cream Full-fat yoghurt Cheese e.g. Stilton, Cheddar, cream cheese Evaporated or condensed milk Imitation cream Excess eggs
	Small amounts from next column	Margarine labelled 'high in polyunsaturates' Corn oil, sunflower oil, soya oil, safflower oil, rapeseed oil, olive oil		All margarines, shortenings, and oils not labelled 'high in monounsaturates and polyunsaturates' Butter, lard, suet, and dripping Vegetable oil or margarine of unknown origin
Other foods	Jelly (low sugar) Sorbet Fat-free homemade soups Low-fat, low-sugar yoghurt Low-fat natural yoghurt	Pastry, puddings, cakes, biscuits, sauces, etc. made with wholemeal flour and fat or oil as above	Packet soups	Pastries, puddings, cakes, and sauces made with whole milk and fat or oil as above Suet dumplings or puddings Ice cream Cream soups

Table 8.6 cont'd.

Eat regularly	Eat in moderation	Avoid eating
Marmite, Bovril, chutneys, and pickles Sugar-free artificial sweeteners Small amounts of low-sugar jam or marmalade	Fish and meat pastes. (thin spread 2–3 times a week) Jelly	Chocolate spreads Chocolate, toffees, fudge butterscotch Carob chocolate Coconut bars
Tea, coffee, mineral water, fruit juices (unsweetened)	Boiled sweets Low-calorie squashes	Sweetened drinks Malted milk or hot chocolate drinks made with skimmed milk / Whole milk drinks Cream-based liqueurs
Herbs, spices, Tabasco, Worcestershire sauce, soy sauce, lemon juice	Homemade dressings and low-fat mayonnaise made with suitable oils	'Low-fat' or 'low-calorie' mayonnaises and dressings. Parmesan cheese / Ordinary or cream dressings and mayonnaises

Eat regularly — Choose from this group daily.
Eat in moderation — Moderate amounts 2–3 times per week.
treat — Moderate amounts once a week or less.

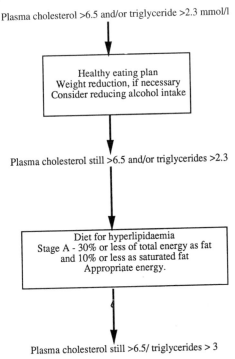

Plasma cholesterol >6.5 and/or triglyceride >2.3 mmol/l

Healthy eating plan
Weight reduction, if necessary
Consider reducing alcohol intake

Plasma cholesterol still >6.5 and/or triglycerides >2.3

Diet for hyperlipidaemia
Stage A - 30% or less of total energy as fat
and 10% or less as saturated fat
Appropriate energy.

Plasma cholesterol still >6.5/ triglycerides > 3

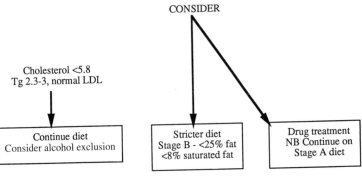

CONSIDER

Cholesterol <5.8
Tg 2.3-3, normal LDL

Continue diet
Consider alcohol exclusion

Stricter diet
Stage B - <25% fat
<8% saturated fat

Drug treatment
NB Continue on
Stage A diet

Fig. 8.1 Plan for stepwise dietary management of hyperlipidaemia.
Note: Actual lipid levels will depend on patients' overall CHD risk.

hyperlipidaemia, or familial combined or remnant hyperlipidaemia. As a general rule drug therapy should not be considered until maximal response to dietary change has been achieved. This often takes several months. If patients who are expected to respond to diet do not respond adequately, then their diet should be reviewed and they may need to reduce the number and frequency of the foods they have been having from the 'in moderation' column.

It is important to point out that the diet recommended for hyperlipidaemia is appropriate for the general population and as such is suitable for other family members who may not have the condition. It is very similar to the diet recommended for people with diabetes (though in those requiring insulin, all carbohydrate will need to be distributed appropriately during the day) and for people with many gastrointestinal diseases. It is only rarely in conflict with other sets of dietary recommendations.

If sensibly planned the diet should be adequate in all nutrients, minerals, and vitamins. Indeed intake may well be higher than on the initial higher fat diet. However, calcium intake may need to be specifically considered, particularly in women. Low-fat diary products contain the same amount, or more, calcium than full-fat products and these should be substituted, and their use generally encouraged. Ways to increase absorption of non-haem iron also need to be considered in people, particularly women, reducing their meat intake. Drinking fruit juice or eating fruit with meals is helpful in this respect.

The cost of a different diet is a question often raised by patients, particularly those on low incomes. It is possible to plan a low-fat diet which is no more expensive than a person's usual diet. Vegetables (particularly in season) and pulses are relatively cheap, brown bread is not significantly more expensive than white, and soft mono- or poly-unsaturated margarines are often less expensive than butter. Table 8.7 gives some simple and inexpensive ways to reduce fat in the diet.

Children with hyperlipidaemia need special consideration. In some instances familial hypercholesterolaemia is diagnosed very early in life. Very young children should not be given a very low-fat diet, but from the age of 3 or 4 years general healthy eating is encouraged, with the avoidance of foods containing excessive saturated fat. Dietary recommendations for older children need to take into account the overall nutritional requirements for growth but this is easily achieved within the basic context of a diet low in saturated fat and high in soluble fibre.

For many people with hyperlipidaemia dietary change is initially difficult, but with appropriate teaching the majority realize that the change not only produces a reduction in blood lipids but provides a palatable alternative to the traditional high-fat 'Western diet'.

Table 8.7   Some practical ways to reduce saturated fat in the diet

- Substitute soft polyunsaturated or monounsaturated margarine for butter.
- Use polyunsaturated or monounsaturated oils.
- Use skimmed milk instead of full-cream milk. Avoid cream.
- Replace ordinary hard cheeses with low-fat or reduced-fat varieties, e.g. cottage cheese, quark (skimmed milk soft cheese), Shape, or supermarket's own brands of half-fat cheese.
- Try low-fat yoghurt and skimmed milk cheeses in place of cream, mayonnaise, and salad cream, or use a small quantity of olive oil.
- Choose lean cuts of meat and trim off fat before cooking.
- Eat smaller portions of meat. Extend meat and poultry dishes by using pulses, cereals, and vegetables.
- Eat chicken, turkey, and fish more often as these are lower in fat. Remove all skin and fat from poultry.
- Grill, steam, poach, bake, braise, or casserole instead of frying or roasting with extra fat. Do not use lard.
  To avoid the need to add fat when roasting, wrap food in foil or roasting bags to retain juices and prevent drying out. Meat can be roasted without fat, or cooked on a rack over a pan of hot water.
- Low-fat sauces can be made by mixing flour or cornflour with cold water, skimmed milk, or stock before cooking to thicken.
- Skim off fat from stews and soups by removing it with absorbent kitchen paper or, if the dish is allowed to cool first, the fat could be scooped off with a spoon.
- Be on the look-out for new low-fat or reduced-fat products in the shops. Check labels for fat content and type of fat used in processed foods.
- In addition, eat more fibre rich foods, particularly fruit and vegetables

Summary

People with hyperlipidaemia should alter their calorie intake to enable them to attain their ideal body weight. Saturated fat intake needs to be reduced. This is best achieved by restricting fat in as many contexts as possible and substituting monosaturated and polyunsaturated fat where suitable. Unrefined carbohydrate should replace refined carbohydrate-containing food where possible, the use of pulses should be encouraged, and sugar and alcohol intake may need to be reduced. Consumption of vegetables and fruit should be increased as they are low in fat and are valuable sources of the antioxidant vitamins. Fish may be of value, particularly as a replacement for meat, because of its content of very long chain polyunsaturated fatty acids.

More information is needed, from prospective studies, on the value of specifically increasing vitamin E intake. More data are also needed about factors such as flavanoids in food and their role in the body.

9

Drug treatment of hyperlipidaemia

Many patients with a familial hyperlipidaemia require treatment with drugs in addition to dietary control, as do some patients without an obvious family history. Drug treatment will depend on age, medical history and family history, as well as other factors. However, it should not be commenced until there has been a careful trial of the most rigorous diet appropriate for the particular patient. In addition, even if drug treatment is required, patients must be advised to continue on an appropriate diet. Studies indicate that the effects of drugs and diet are additive.

A number of drugs are currently available for the treatment of hyperlipidaemia (Table 9.1). Some are most suitable for the treatment of raised cholesterol; others are used to lower both cholesterol and triglycerides, or substantially raised triglycerides.

Bile acid sequestrants (cholestyramine and colestipol)

The effectiveness of cholestyramine has been shown in the LRCPPT and STARS (Chapter 4). These drugs are a good treatment for hypercholesterolaemia caused by a high LDL cholesterol. They are anion exchange resins which have their main action in the intestine. The resins complex with bile salts in the intestine and result in their excretion in the faeces, rather than reabsorption and use. This loss means that more bile salts need to be synthesized, and this involves the use of cholesterol (Fig. 9.1). Depletion of cell cholesterol leads to an increase in LDL receptors and LDL removal from the plasma. Constant use of these resins thus results in a lowering of the plasma cholesterol. Total and LDL cholesterol are often reduced by 15–25 per cent, and HDL cholesterol may rise slightly. Triglycerides may, however, rise slightly so these drugs should not be used alone in patients who have a plasma triglyceride above 3 mmol/l, and the effect on plasma triglycerides should be monitored in

Table 9.1   Drug therapy
Note–Availability of preparations may vary in different countries

---

Cholestyramine (Questran and Questran Lite)
   Availability — 4 g sachets, or tin of powder
   Dosage   — 1–6 sachets or scoops/day

Colestipol (Colestid)
   Availability — 5 g sachets
   Dosage   — 1–6 sachets/day

Probucol (Lurselle)
   Availability — 250 mg tablets
   Dosage   — 500 mg twice a day

Bezafibrate (Bezalip)
   Availability — 200 mg tablets
                — 400 mg long-acting preparation (Bezalip mono)
Dosage—200 mg three times a day or 400 mg Bezalip mono/day

Clofibrate (Atromid-S)
   Availability — 500 mg capsules
   Dosage   — 500 mg twice or three times a day

Gemfibrozil (Lopid)
   Availability — 300 mg tablets, 600 mg capsules (Australia)
   Dosage   — 300 mg three or four times a day

Lovastatin (Mevacor)
   Availability — 10, 20, 40 mg tablets
   Dosage   — 20–80 mg

Simvastatin (Zocor)
   Availability — 5, 10, and 20 mg tablets
   Dosage   — 5–40 mg at night

Pravastatin (Lipostat)
   Availability — 10 mg tablets
   Dosage   — 10–40 mg at night

---

anyone with a level exceeding the reference range. The daily dosage of cholestyramine required varies from 4 to 28 g. The resin is packaged in tins or sachets. The sachets contain 4 g of resin. The preparation

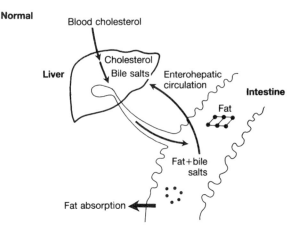

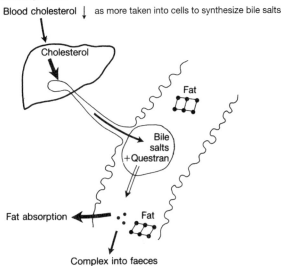

Fig. 9.1 Mechanism of action of cholestyramine.

'Questran Lite' contains only 1 g of other products and is thus less bulky than the original 'Questran'. It should be dissolved in an appropriate quantity of water or juice and shaken to give a good suspension prior to ingestion. A marked glass can be used. The mixture is slightly unpalatable, but the addition of fruit juice usually improves its acceptability. Some people find it convenient and preferable to leave the suspension in the refrigerator for several hours and decant a quantity at appropriate times. Ideas are given in the Appendix for those who dislike taking it. It can also be mixed with cereal, or foods like soup after cooking.

It is wise to start patients on a low dose—one or two sachets a day— and gradually increase if necessary, because flatulence and mild abdominal discomfort sometimes occur. If constipation results then this may be eased by an increase in dietary fibre. Malabsorption is very rare, but when the drug is used in children a folic acid preparation is given. The resins may, however, interfere with the absorption of other drugs, and it is sensible precaution to take other medication at a different time. A few patients, particularly those with pre-existing gastro-intestinal problems, are unable to tolerate the dose of cholestyramine required. It is then sensible to try another drug, or a combination of medications with only a small dose of resin.

Combinations of resins in small doses and submaximal doses of HMGcoA reductase inhibitors are being used by some physicians.

Probucol

In the recommended dose of 500 mg b.d. probucol gives a variable response, but it may lower the plasma LDL cholesterol by 10–15 per cent when used in conjunction with an appropriate diet. Its maximal effect occurs after 1–3 months treatment, but it appears to be less effective than cholestyramine and it has the disadvantages of reducing HDL cholesterol levels as well as LDL. The specific mode of action is unclear, although it probably enhances removal of LDL from the circulation, and it does usually reduce the size of xanthomas. Oral absorption is low, but appears to be more uniform when the drug is taken with food. Accumulation in adipose tissue occurs, with the result that the drug may be present in the body for months after the last dose.

Tolerance of probucol is good, with only occasional patients reporting nausea and flatulence. It can, however, cause prolongation of QT interval and could potentiate arrythmias, so it should be used cautiously in patients with ischaemic heart disease. The safety of the drug in children or during pregnancy has not been established. Despite these factors, some interest in this preparation has remained because it has marked anti-oxidant properties. A couple of studies evaluating this are in progress.

Fibric acid derivatives

There are a number of fibrates licenced for use in different countries. They included fenofibrate, clofibrate, bezafibrate, and gemfibrozil. They act by several mechanisms, and their main effect is to reduce VLDL cholesterol. This causes a fall in plasma cholesterol and triglyceride levels.

Clofibrate

The WHO clofibrate trial showed that the treatment of hyperlipidaemic men with this drug reduced their morbidity from myocardial infarction. There was, however, an increase in deaths from other causes and in the incidence of gallstones. Owing to this it is not commonly recommended, although in remnant hyperlipidaemia it may have a dramatic effect, better than that of other fibrates, and in this context the benefit is likely to outweigh any risks.

Bezafibrate

This drug is an analogue of clofibrate and has been a first-line drug in the treatment of familial combined hyperlipidaemia. It is also of value in patients with familial hypercholesterolaemia—both in those who are unable to tolerate cholestyramine, and as an additional agent in those with inadequate response. Bezafibrate is given as 200 mg t.d.s. or as a once-daily 400 mg preparation, Bezalip-mono. It reduces total cholesterol, particularly LDL cholesterol, decreases the LDL/HDL cholesterol ratio and also reduces plasma triglycerides. Effectiveness in this respect has been noted in diabetics, and it may also help to reduce blood glucose.

Gemfibrozil

This drug is another analogue which has similar properties. The large Helsinki Heart trial has shown the beneficial effects of lipid lowering using this drug (Chapter 4). There was a 34 per cent reduction in coronary events associated with mean falls in cholesterol, LDL cholesterol, and triglycerides of 8 per cent, 9 per cent, and 40 per cent, respectively. The incidence of side-effects was not appreciably different from placebo. It is not currently available as a single daily dose. It is effective in improving the lipid profile in diabetics.

Side-effects

The incidence of side-effects from bezafibrate and gemfibrozil is low. Those most frequently experienced are gastrointestinal, such as nausea and a feeling of fullness, although occasionally more severe upset and abdominal pain have been reported. Elevated liver-function tests are seen in 0.1–2 per cent of patients, but often resolve despite continuation of the drug. Intermittent measurement of liver-function tests are, nevertheless, recommended. Impotence may sometimes occur, although this seems more common on bezafibrate than gemfibrozil. Myositis, such as was occasionally seen with clofibrate, occurs very rarely and usually when combinations of drugs are being used. The drugs are contra-indicated during pregnancy and in people with severe renal or hepatic disease. There is a little information available about their safety and effectiveness in less severe renal disease and nephrotic syndrome, but the dose must usually be reduced. The fibrates may potentiate the action of warfarin and patients requiring therapy with these two drugs must be carefully monitored. Unlike clofibrate, bezafibrate and gemfibrozil have little effect on the lithogenic index of bile, and are probably not associated with a marked increase in the incidence of gallstones.

In some people with combined hyperlipidaemia the use of fibrates may increase LDL cholesterol, although reducing total cholesterol and triglyceride. If this occurs then a small dose of bile acid sequestrant can be added.

Nicotinic acid derivatives

These preparations reduce VLDL and LDL synthesis and thus cause a fall in LDL cholesterol and triglyceride levels. The effect tends to be variable when the medication is used alone, but in some patients, particularly those with familial combined hyperlipidaemia, they provide an additional benefit when a single drug has insufficient effect. In the Coronary Drug Project, patients taking niacin had a reduction in CHD deaths at 15-year follow-up.

The effectiveness of combination therapy in reducing CHD has been demonstrated in secondary prevention trials. It has also been noted that nicotinic acid can reduce Lp(a) levels.

Patients often experience flushing and a sensation of warmth after taking these preparations, and treatment is best started with a low dose,

given several times a day with food, and increased gradually to a dose
of 2–3 grams per day. The flushing is mediated by prostaglandins and
can be reduced by low doses of aspirin. Nicotinic acid itself often has
unacceptable side-effects, but patients may tolerate analogues such as
nicofuranose, acipimox or inositol nicotinate, although these may give
less lipid lowering. Gout and abnormalities of liver function may sometimes occur.

Maxepa

The omega-3 fatty acids in fish oil may be of use in some patients with
severe hypertriglyceridaemia, but more data are needed, particularly in
comparison with other treatments. The effect on LDL cholesterol seems
to depend on the dose, and at low doses LDL may actually rise,
although VLDL falls. The value of the changes it can cause in the clotting mechanism, platelet function, and blood rheology, and its interaction with any other drugs remain to be shown. In diabetics,
triglycerides may be reduced, but some reports suggest that blood
glucose control may deteriorate. Antioxidants have to be added to these
very unsaturated fatty acids to avoid the formation of toxic oxidation
products.

HMGCoA reductase inhibitors

The HMGcoA reductase inhibitors are a first line treatment for patients
with familial hypercholesterolaemia and are increasingly used in
people with hypercholesterolaemia refractory to conventional treatment. These drugs include lovostatin, simvastatin, and pravastatin.
They are chemicals which act within the cells to block the action of
HMGCoA reductase, an enzyme responsible for the synthesis of
cholesterol. In practice, when the cholesterol supply to the cell from the
plasma is reduced by drugs such as cholestyramine, the endogenous
synthesis of cholesterol may increase. This resets the balance somewhat with the net result that plasma cholesterol does not fall to the
extent expected. By blocking cholesterol synthesis a greater lipid-
lowering effect can be achieved.

These drugs often give very effective reductions in cholesterol, with
reductions in LDL cholesterol of 20–45 per cent. Combination with

bile acid sequestrants may improve this further. They have little effect on triglyceride or HDL levels, although a few studies have shown slight benefits. Long-term safety data are still awaited. Abnormalities of liver function tests sometimes occur and this needs further evaluation. The plasma creatine kinase level may also rise transiently. Clinical experience indicates that combinations of reductase inhibitors and cyclosporin, fibrates, or nicotinic acid may increase the risk of myopathy. No deficiencies of cholesterol-based steroid hormones, such as cortisol or the sex hormones, have been described during treatment. HMGCoA reductase inhibitors are potentially teratogenic so their use will generally have to be confined to men, and women who are post-menopausal, surgically sterile, or taking adequate precautions to prevent pregnancy. Use in children is not currently advised by the manufacturers, but they have been used in adolescents with FH by a few clinicians.

Figure 9.2 shows a plan for the treatment of a person with hyperlipidaemia.

Patients with homozygous familial hypercholesterolaemia seldom achieve acceptable cholesterol levels, even with maximal drug therapy. Additional measures may then be considered in these patients.

Plasma exchange/plasmaphoresis

This form of treatment is sometimes used in patients with very high cholesterol levels, such as those with homozygous familial hypercholesterolaemia. The treatment temporarily reduces the cholesterol, but the procedure has to be repeated every few weeks. Plasma replacement also has potential risks. Several types of specific apheresis have been developed which specifically remove LDL and VLDL and do not require plasma infusion, but these are very expensive and are under continued evaluation.

Surgical procedures

Ileal bypass has been performed in a few patients with severe hypercholesterolaemia resistant to drug treatment, and in some patients with homozygous familial hypercholesterolaemia. The result of this surgical procedure is a reduction in the reabsorption of bile acids, which usually

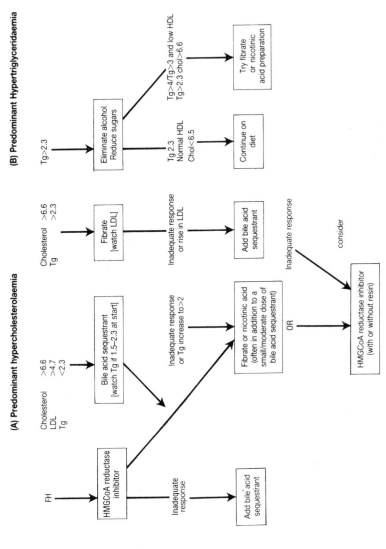

Fig. 9.2 Flow diagram of the suggested treatment of primary hyperlipidaemia in a young to middle-aged adult.
Note: Lipid levels at which treatment is suggested depend on overall risk determined by assessment of other risk factors.

occurs as part of the enterohepatic circulation. Unfortunately the opera-
tion frequently has unwanted side-effects, including severe diarrhoea
and metabolic disturbances, and is rarely performed in most countries.
Its success in reducing lipid levels and the incidence of CHD has,
however, been shown in the PROCAM study.

Summary

Currently, bile acid sequestrants and the HMGCoA reductase inhibitors
are generally regarded as first-line drug treatment for hypercholesterolaemia due to high LDL cholesterol levels. The two drugs
can be used together.

Bezafibrate, gemfibrozil, and nicotinic acid are first-line drug treatments for patients with raised cholesterol and triglyceride levels, and
for those with significant primary hypertriglyceridaemia. Addition of
cholestyramine may sometimes be needed if the LDL rises. A small
number of patients will need a combination of two drug types.

Many patients with hyperlipidaemia have a very satisfactory
decrease in plasma cholesterol when undergoing dietary control in
combination with single drug treatment. Some patients do, however,
require additional drug treatment. The reasons for long-term treatment
and its importance must be emphasized to the patients, as compliance
may be reduced when they do not feel any immediate benefit.

10

Overview of the familial hyperlipidaemias and patient treatment: other aspects of management

Familial hypercholesterolaemia

Incidence	Approximately 1 in 500
Inheritance	Autosomal dominant
Cause	Genetic defect. Usually reduced number of LDL receptors
Effect	High plasma LDL cholesterol; very high risk CHD
Clinical signs	
	Tendon xanthomas
	Xanthelasmas
	Early corneal arcus
Treatment	
(a) Diet	Low saturated fat diet, increase in P:S ratio, high fibre, appropriate calories to attain ideal body weight
(b) Drugs	HMGCoA reductase inhibitor or bile acid sequestrant
(c) Reduce other CHD risk factors	

Follow-up as appropriate
Screen family

Familial combined hyperlipidaemia

Incidence	Approximately 1 in 300
Inheritance	Likely to be autosomal dominant
Effect	High plasma VLDL cholesterol (cholesterol and triglyceride raised)
	High risk premature CHD

Treatment
- (a) Diet   Low saturated fat diet, increase in P+M:S ratio, high fibre, appropriate calories to attain ideal body weight
- (b) Drugs   Fibric acid derivative, perhaps with a small dose of a bile acid sequestrant if LDL cholesterol raised
- (c) Reduced other CHD risk factors

Follow-up as appropriate

Screen family members >18 years. Tell parents about reminding younger children to be tested at 18 and 25 years

Remnant hyperlipidaemia

Incidence	1 in 10 000
Inheritance	?
Cause	Apo E2/E2 plus another primary or secondary factor
Effect	High risk CHD
	High risk peripheral vascular disease
Clinical signs	Tuboeruptive xanthomas

Treatment
- (a) Identification of any secondary factor and treatment
- (b) Diet
- (c) Drug treatment with a fibrate if necessary

Familial hypertriglyceridaemia

Incidence	Approximately 1 in 1000
Inheritance	Probably autosomal dominant
Clinical signs	Eruptive xanthomas if triglyceride concentrations markedly raised
Effect	Risk of pancreatitis if concentrations exceed 20 mmol/l

Treatment

(a) Secondary factors such as diet, weight, glucose intolerance, and alcohol intake are often very important and treatment of these factors may reduce levels significantly

(b) Drug treatment—if levels remain elevated (generally >4 mmol/l), especially if the HDL cholesterol is low. Fibrates are often effective. Fish oils may be useful.

Genetic counselling

If one parent has familial hypercholesterolaemia there is a 50 per cent chance that any children will inherit the gene and have the condition. The risk is probably the same in familial combined hyperlipidaemia.

Heterozygous familial hypercholesterolaemia can often be diagnosed at birth, although testing is often postponed until the child is older. The wishes of the parents as to the timing of the diagnosis in children should be considered. Testing between the ages of four and six is probably sensible. Interpretation of the results should be performed by someone with experience in diagnosis in children as the reference range is very different in young children (see Chapter 6). Even then it may not be possible to confirm or exclude the condition in all children. A high level can be confirmative, but a borderline or high 'normal range' level may be found, particularly when the family are on a low-fat diet. In these cases repeat testing should be arranged a year or two later.

In families with familial combined hyperlipidaemia testing should not be performed until the offspring are in their late teens or early twenties, as the lipids are seldom raised in childhood. Even at this age the disorder may not be manifest or the levels may only be marginally elevated. Follow-up and repeat testing should therefore be offered in the mid or late twenties.

The revelation that there is a serious genetic disorder in the family can be absolutely devastating, even for unaffected members. A parent with premature cardiovascular disease needs reassurance that with effective treatment the prognosis for their child is likely to be much better than their own. Feelings of guilt that they have passed on illness on to their children may remain, however. In the unlikely case of two individuals with familial hypercholesterolaemia marrying then there is a 1 in 2 chance that any child will inherit one gene and have heterozygous familial hypercholesterolaemia and a 1 in 4 chance that they will inherit two genes resulting in the very severe homozygous form.

Treatment of other risk factors

The importance of risk factors other than hyperlipidaemia were discussed in Chapter 3.

Smoking

Cigarette smoking causes an increased incidence of CHD, with a relatively greater risk in people under the age of 50. It acts synergistically with risk factors such as hypercholesterolaemia. There is evidence that smoking may adversely affect lipid levels by slightly reducing the plasma HDL and the HDL/LDL ratio. It may also increase the susceptibility of lipids to oxidation, and have adverse effects on vessel tone and endothelial function. Surveys show that a large percentage of smokers would like to give up and feel that advice from their doctors would provide an incentive. All patients who smoke should ideally receive personal counselling including information on the hazards, the potential benefits of discontinuing, advice on ways to stop and to cope with the problems, and a target. Fear of a small weight gain is not a justifiable excuse for continuing to smoke, as in most cases even a 5–10 kg weight gain is a lesser health risk than smoking 20 cigarettes a day and with appropriate advice weight gain should be much less. Nicotine chewing gum, acupuncture, hypnosis, and group therapy can be helpful.

Some patients find it difficult to stop smoking completely while changing their diet, particularly if this involves calorie reduction. Encouraging patients to realize which cigarettes are smoked at 'habit times' and to initially stop these while implementing the diet may prove more acceptable, and improve compliance. Various programmes aimed at helping people quit smoking can be very successful. Particularly for those without CHD, nicotine chewing gum or patches are sometimes useful, and new substances without nicotine are available.

Hypertension

The combination of hypertension and hyperlipidaemia is relatively common. In a very few individuals treatment with thiazides or beta blockers may cause an increase in plasma triglycerides, so it is probably prudent to check the plasma lipids before starting antihypertensive treatment, if possible.

● *Diuretics.*   Thiazide diuretics tend to increase the production of triglyceride-rich VLDL from the liver. This may cause an increase in plasma triglyceride levels in some patients, but the rise is usually clinically insignificant. In a very few patients, however, there is a marked rise in plasma triglycerides to a level which could constitute a risk for vascular problems or pancreatitis. The effects on lipids may be dose dependent and lower doses may give marginally less antihypertensive effect but may not affect lipid metabolism. Indapamide (at 2.5 mg/day) does not have adverse effects on lipid levels. Short-term administration of frusemide may increase cholesterol and triglycerides, and reduce HDL; longer-term therapy appears only to affect HDL. Spironolactone and amiloride have no adverse effects.

● *β-Blockers.*   The effect of different β-blockers appears to be variable, although the trend is probably similar. Several studies have shown that plasma triglycerides are increased slightly on long-term treatment; the greatest rise occurring with the non-selective β-antagonist propranolol. Propranolol also reduces HDL cholesterol and increases the total cholesterol/HDL cholesterol ratio. Other β-blockers are there-fore preferable to propranolol in patients with hyperlipidaemia. The effect of the selective β-blockers is small, and it is usual to leave well-controlled hyperlipidaemic patients on them. β-adrenergic blocking agents with partial intrinsic sympathomimetic activity such as acebutalol and pindolol are usually lipid neutral, as is labetolol. Celiprolol actually decreases LDL and triglycerides and can increase HDL cholesterol.

● *α-Blockers.*   Total cholesterol and triglyceride concentrations appear to be unaffected or to fall on prazosin and HDL may increase. The same appears true for indormin and doxazosin.

● *Calcium antagonists.*   Drugs such as nifedepine and diltiazem do not increase plasma lipids. It has been reported that nicardipine decreases triglycerides, and nimodipine decreases cholesterol.

● *Nitrates and angiotensin converting enzyme inhibitors.*   We are not aware of any adverse effect of these drugs on plasma lipids. Most of the drugs that have been studied have been shown to be lipid-neutral.

Now that more drugs are available for the treatment of hypertension, it would seem sensible, in the future, to try drugs without a potential adverse effect on plasma lipids in patients with hyperlipidaemia. It is unfortunate in these times of cost restriction that these are often the more expensive drugs.

Lack of exercise

An increase in activity, particularly walking and swimming, is likely to benefit most people, especially those with a sedentary lifestyle. It can assist weight reduction and it may, independently, cause a small increase in HDL cholesterol, particularly HDL_2. In diabetics, exercise also increases insulin sensitivity. Exercise may also be of psychological benefit and this may positively affect compliance to diet. The degree of exertion should be increased gradually, particularly in those who already have CHD, and the exercise should be performed regularly. Table 10.1 show the type of benefits which appear to be attainable at different intensities of exercise.

Obesity

This may predispose to a number of medical problems which include glucose intolerance and hyperlipidaemia. Some patients who are only moderately overweight (10 per cent) may show a marked reduction in plasma lipids on weight reduction. Figure 10.1 gives an idea of the range of desirable weight by height, and a more detailed guide to ideal body weights is given in Table 8.1 (p. 81). The body mass index (BMI)

Table 10.1   Effects of exercise

Parameter improved	Frequency of exercise needed	Intensity	Time
Flexibility	Daily	Comfortable tension	10 seconds/ stretch
Muscular strength	Twice weekly	According to ability	
Cardiovascular endurance	Three times weekly	65–80% maximum heart rate	20–30 minutes
TG/HDL levels	Four times weekly	50–60% maximum heart rate	40–60 minutes

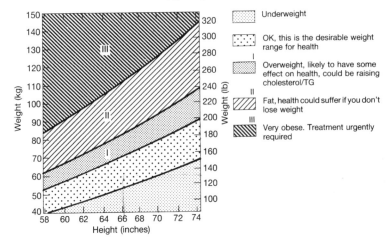

Fig. 10.1 Ideal weight. Being overweight tends to raise blood cholesterol as well as causing other problems. Therefore it is essential to achieve and maintain an ideal weight. This depends on sex, build, and so on. (From Garrow, J.S. (1988). *Obesity and related diseases*. Churchill Livingstone.)

is used to assess obesity. This index is calculated as the person's weight in kilograms divided by their height^2 in metres^2. A BMI greater than 25 indicates that someone is overweight, and an index of 30 that they are seriously obese. The risk of obesity is particularly great if associated with a high waist: hip ratio.

Planning a realistic weight loss programme and follow-up of patients trying to lose weight is important. Many overweight individuals find that joining a slimming club provides encouragement and support.

Oestrogen and progestogen usage

Much has been written about the effects of various oral contraceptive preparations on plasma lipid levels. In general, oestrogens tend to increase plasma triglyceride levels and reduce plasma cholesterol, and may increase HDL. Progestogens tend to lower HDL cholesterol levels, although the effect does depend on the type of progestogen: progestogens with androgenic antioestrogenic activity, such as levonorgestrel, appear to have the greatest effect. The overall effect on plasma lipids depends on the relative dose of the constituents.

Oral contraceptives

The advisability of oral contraceptive usage depends on several factors and must be assessed for each woman. Much of the epidemiological data are still based on long-term use of older preparations. Low-dose, triphasic preparations or a preparation containing a progestogen with weak androgenic activity, such as Marvelon, are likely to be most suitable for those who wish to use this method of contraception, as they have little overall effect on plasma lipids. For older women who smoke it would be expected that there may be some increased risk for combined oral contraceptive use, as in normolipidaemic women. Weak androgenic progestogen-only pills can be considered.

The use of postmenopausal hormone replacement must also be considered carefully. A number of retrospective case-control studies suggest a reduction in relative risk of CHD with use of hormone replacement therapy. Most women included in these studies were, however, on oestrogen alone rather than the 'opposed' therapy with intermittent or continuous progestogens—which is the form of replacement currently prescribed for women who have a uterus. The effects on lipid levels do depend on the preparations used but are less than those seen with combined oral contraceptives. The so-called 'natural' oestrogens would tend to improve the lipid profile, and with sequential progestogen use the lipid levels can vary at different times in the cycle. Reported effects of oestrogen implants and patches are inconsistent. There are, however, few data on hyperlipidaemic women using combined preparations and the effects may be different in those with a disorder of lipid metabolism. Measurement of lipids after a couple of months' usage would seem sensible in these women. Use in women who are symptomatic or at high risk of osteoporosis seems very appropriate. More data would be desirable for other women.

Effects of some other medications

Patients with CHD may be prescribed a number of different types of medication both for their CHD and for intercurrent diseases. The possible effects of any drugs on plasma lipids and any interaction with lipid-lowering drugs should be considered. For example, several case reports have indicated that amiodarone can increase plasma LDL cholesterol. Warfarin may increase cholesterol and triglycerides slightly. Post-transplantation elevations of total and LDL cholesterol are observed with cyclosporin, probably due to the fact that the drug inhibits an enzyme involved in the formation of bile salts from cholesterol.

Cholestyramine may interfere with the absorption of other drugs administered at the same time, and it is preferable for them to be given at least an hour apart. Cholestyramine and the fibrates may potentiate the action of warfarin, so careful monitoring of the prothrombin time is needed in people on warfarin and the dose may sometimes need to be reduced slightly.

Psychology

When an individual is found to have hyperlipidaemia, particularly a familial hyperlipidaemia, it is often a great shock. Suddenly they are advised to make alterations which may completely change their lifestyle. This often seems a very difficult task, particularly if they feel well and the raised lipids have been found during screening. Obviously each person is an individual in his/her knowledge, perception, needs, and aims. Motivation to make changes varies, although it is often high in those with a familial condition, who have seen relatives die young from CHD, and in those who have had a myocardial infarction. Intrinsic motivation is more powerful than extrinsic motivation so patients need to be allowed to feel that they are 'in control' and have responsibility for their own health. Motivation in many people increases with success, and for these people it is important that the lifestyle changes needed are structured into steps which are achievable and ordered logically. The individual's previous health beliefs need to be considered as they may affect or interfere with the acquisition and application of new knowledge. One aspect of this is their interpretation of previous information which they have been given about their condition. Checking this and correcting any misconceptions may be time well spent. Incorrect beliefs about health matters which have been held for a long time or which are the opinion of respected friends may be very difficult to modify. Encouraging people to ask questions and to work out arguments and plans for themselves, although time consuming, is likely to produce positive long-term results. The information and explanations provided often have more impact and are more readily remembered if the person feels they are directly relevant to them, rather than being rather general facts. Relatives of individuals with hyperlipidaemia sometimes ignore suggestions from affected relatives that doctors have advised blood testing. This may be because of fear of a positive result. The point has to be stressed that if they are tested then they can be offered appropriate treatment to reduce the risks.

Important aspects of the patient/health professional interviews thus include:

(1) eliciting the patient's health beliefs and what they have already been told about their condition and their interpretation of this;
(2) countering misinformation and inappropriate negative attitudes, and reinforcing positive attitudes; giving the patient more information;
(3) planning with the patient an appropriate course of action, taking into consideration the individual's circumstances;
(4) eliciting degree of motivation and how to reinforce positive changes;
(5) providing appropriate follow-up.

Section III

Screening

11

Population and high-risk strategies in coronary heart disease prevention

Much has been written about the advantages and disadvantages of the two risk-reduction strategies for the prevention of premature coronary heart disease. One is aimed at the entire population and the other is targeted at high-risk individuals. Both are essential in any serious attempt to reduce premature CHD in high-risk populations. This chapter describes the two approaches and emphasizes how they are linked.

Population strategy

The population strategy is based on the recognition that where CHD is common, the majority of cases occur among those with moderately elevated levels of cholesterol and other risk factors. Figure 11.1 shows how an individual's risk increases with increasing levels of serum cholesterol, but that most of the CHD cases attributable to the cholesterol-associated risk do not occur from the few at high risk but from the large numbers exposed to a lesser risk. The population strategy aims to improve nutritional habits (and other health-oriented behaviour) so that the average level of cholesterol in the population falls. As there is no important threshold in the relation between cholesterol level and CHD (see Chapter 2) this will result in a population at less risk of CHD. If this is carried out in conjunction with a reduction in other CHD risk factors, a substantial reduction in the epidemic of premature CHD might be expected.

The principles of dietary change which might be recommended for the whole population are similar to the initial guidelines for individuals with hyperlipidaemia described in Chapter 8, although they are usually rather less restrictive.

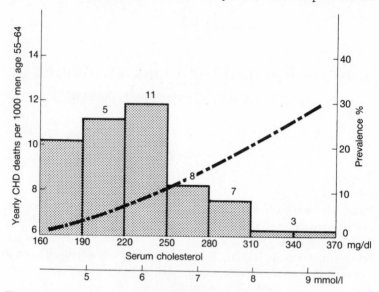

Fig. 11.1 Prevalence distribution of serum cholesterol, and CHD mortality risk (— · — · — · —). (From WHO Technical Report 670, 1982.) Numbers over column represent attributable deaths/1000 men per ten years.

These are, basically:

(1) control of overweight;
(2) reduction of saturated fatty acids to 10 per cent or less of total energy;
(3) increased consumption of soluble fibre;
(4) partial replacement of saturated fatty acids by mono- and poly-unsaturated fatty acids;
(5) restriction of dietary cholesterol to 300 mg, or less, per day.

The difference between the average recommendation and the diet typically eaten in most Western countries is given in Fig. 11.2.

The nutritional guidelines issued by various national and international organizations differ both in emphasis and in the quantities recommended. However if the recent British Dietary Reference Values were to be adopted (Fig. 11.2) it is possible to predict (from various published studies) the effect on the mean serum cholesterol of the population. If there was full compliance with these recommendations the mean cholesterol level found in 25–59 year old men and women in

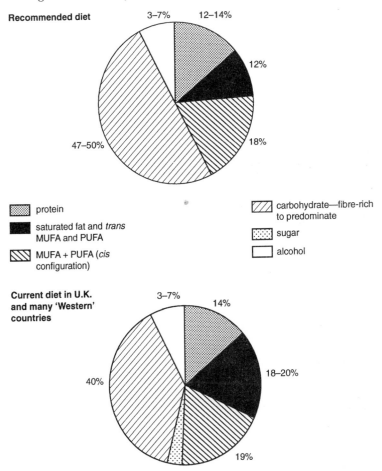

Fig. 11.2 Comparison of UK diet and diet recommended for the population.

the British National Lipid Screening Project would be expected to be reduced by approximately 12 per cent from 5.9 to 5.2 mmol/l.

Table 11.1 shows the percentage of people who currently have cholesterol levels exceeding certain selected cut-off points, and the effect of various reductions in cholesterol. A mean reduction of 12 per cent, predicted to result from full compliance with the dietary reference values, would leave an expected 38 per cent of the population with a plasma

Table 11.1   Percentage of UK population aged 25–59 with plasma cholesterol above certain limits and predicted effect of adopting moderate dietary recommendations

Plasma cholesterol (mmol/l)	>6.5	>5.7	>5.2
Prevalence study 1984/5	23	45	63
Mean reduction of 7–9% 1	12	30	50
Mean reduction of 12%	6	23	38
Mean reduction of 17%	3	12	20

[1] incomplete compliance with dietary reference values;
[2] complete compliance with dietary reference values;
[3] complete compliance to WHO recommendations.

cholesterol greater than 5.2 mmol/l (a level associated with some degree of risk) and an expected 6 per cent with hyperlipidaemia (level >6.5 mmol/l). Adherence to the more restrictive WHO dietary recommendations would lead to a fall of 17 per cent in serum cholesterol, and only 20 per cent of the population would continue to have undesirable levels and 3 per cent would have high levels. In the more likely situation of incomplete dietary compliance with the dietary reference values the proportion with appreciable hyperlipidaemia would be relatively high (see Table 11.1). All these calculations are made on the assumption that dietary change is isocaloric. Moderate success in reducing the prevalence and extent of obesity would substantially increase the fall in cholesterol, but it is not possible to say by precisely how much.

Individual or high-risk strategy

It is clear from the above discussion that even with a high level of compliance with appropriate dietary recommendations, a substantial proportion of the population will continue to be at high risk of CHD because of high levels of cholesterol. Of particular importance is the fact that virtually all individuals with familial hypercholesterolaemia, the majority with familial combined hyperlipidaemia and remnant hyperlipoproteinaemia, and some people with other forms of hyperlipidaemia, do not show an adequate response, even with full compliance to the kind of dietary recommendations suitable for the general public. For them a more stringent diet (see Chapter 8) and often drug therapy are necessary, and appropriate follow-up is essential. A high-risk strategy is thus required to complement the population strategy so that these people can be identified and given individual care.

It has been suggested that selective screening of those with various 'risk attributes' for blood lipids will enable the majority of people with marked hyperlipidaemia to be detected. Tables 11.2 and 11.3 show the proportions of those with cholesterol levels greater than 6.5 or 8.0 mmol/l who would be found if various criteria were used to determine which people should be screened. The two most helpful criteria are a family history of CHD and obesity, each of which identifies roughly half of those with raised levels of cholesterol. Using all the criteria listed, it is possible to detect about 78 per cent of those with raised levels, but in order to do so it would be necessary to screen 66 per cent of the population. It is perhaps surprising that a family history of CHD and, in particular, a family history of premature CHD, is not more helpful as a predictor of raised cholesterol levels in the general population, although it is a better predictor of familial hypercholesterolaemia, which, as mentioned before, carries a particularly high risk. One possible reason for a lower than expected pick-up related to family

Table 11.2 Detection of hyperlipidaemic individuals according to criteria used for screening

		Cholesterol >6.5 mmol/l	
Screening criterion	Percentage of population with this attribute	Percentage found using this criterion	% of all people with cholesterol >6.5
Family history CHD	38	29	44[1]
Corneal arcus	6	40	10
Xanthomas	3	37	4
Obesity (BMI >25)	43	32	54
Hypertension	12	38	19
Either family history or obesity	64	29	74
Any of the above	66	29	78

[1] If one screens everyone with a family history of CHD, one will find 29 per cent of people to have a cholesterol > 6.5 mmol/l. This represents 44 per cent of the total population who have a cholesterol above this.

Table 11.3 Detection of hypercholesterolaemia (>8.0 mmol/l) using various selective screening criteria

Screening criterion	Hypercholesterolaemia (>8.0 mmol/l) detected
Family history	50%
Family history CHD under age 50	12%
Corneal arcus	13%
Xanthomas or xanthelasma	5%
Obesity (BMI > 25)	54%
Hypertension (BP 160/90)	21%
Family history or obesity	77%
Any of the above criteria	81%
None of the above criteria	19%

history is that when inheritance of the raised lipid levels occurs via the mother she may die from other causes before CHD manifests itself. This is because women with hyperlipidaemia have a lower risk of CHD compared with men and it tends to occur later in life.

A number of options are available to detect those with markedly raised cholesterol levels and these are outlined below.

General population screening

A quarter of the population with hyperlipidaemia would not fit into any of the categories suggested for special screening. Clearly the only way one could find all those at particular risk would be by general population screening. This has been recommended in some countries, but while this might be the ultimate goal there are several major problems which need to be overcome:

1. At present, lipid measurements are usually made on a venous blood sample in a routine laboratory. This analysis takes time and the administration of such a screening service is a fairly complicated procedure. Equipment is available for the measurement of cholesterol and triglyceride to be made on a finger-prick blood sample.

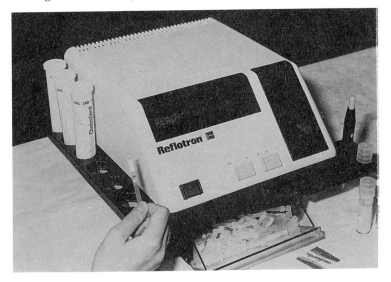

Fig. 11.3 'Reflotron' dry chemistry analyser.

Machines such as the 'Reflotron' (Fig. 11.3) are, however, costly and, although relatively robust, must be used carefully and with consideration of quality control. Smaller and cheaper devices are becoming available. Cost–benefit calculations are rather difficult, but the availability of a quick and cheap method of measurement can improve the balance.

2. Although there is clear evidence for the benefit of cholesterol lowering, there are few data to show how many of those shown to have raised cholesterol levels in routine screening will accept the dietary advice (and sometimes drug treatment) necessary to reduce their blood lipids.

3. If general population screening is undertaken, it is imperative that this be done in an environment in which overall cardiovascular risk assessment can be made. Recommendations concerning blood lipids can only be made with the knowledge of other cardiovascular risk factors.

4. Appropriately qualified and trained health professionals should be available to give advice regarding risk modifications.

5. Facilities for follow-up must be available.

Case finding

It is now an accepted part of good clinical practice (although it is still
not universally applied) that people with certain characteristics should
be screened for hyperlipidaemia.

Screening those with a family history of CHD and those who are
appreciably overweight will identify a reasonable proportion of those
with raised lipid levels. The presence of premature corneal arcus or
xanthomas are relatively specific indicators of hyperlipidaemia and
should prompt blood lipid measurement, even though they will only
identify a small proportion of hyperlipidaemic individuals. The presence of other risk factors for CHD (such as hypertension or diabetes) is
also an indication for screening, not only because such people may
have elevated lipid levels, but also because the coexistence of more
than one risk factor appreciably increases CHD risk. Anyone who is
sufficiently interested to ask for his cholesterol to be measured should
be given the opportunity since such people are likely to be well motivated to implement dietary changes or to comply with drug therapy
should this be necessary.

Development to opportunistic screening

Opportunistic screening for cardiovascular risk factors is now almost as
widely accepted as case finding. This involves offering screening to all
who attend general practitioners' surgeries regardless of the purpose of
the visit. Since 90 per cent of people in countries such as Britain,
Australia, and New Zealand attend their doctors' surgeries at least once
over a 5-year period, this would enable a large proportion of the population to be screened. Although many young and middle-aged men do
not attend in this period, they can often be contacted via their wives.
Such a scheme has been successfully introduced into many general
practices. Where there is enthusiasm, over 90 per cent of people have
accepted the offer of screening when it is made directly at the surgery,
despite the fact that it involves returning for the measurement of blood
lipids and assessment of other cardiovascular risk factors. In general it
is usually appropriate to screen in the 25–60-year age group, although
screening individuals for suspected familial hypercholesterolaemia may
be undertaken in childhood. Most patients identified should be handled
in general practice as the majority will respond if they adhere to an
appropriate lipid-lowering diet and for many others the drug therapy is

relatively straightforward. A specialist clinic will, nevertheless, be needed to deal with difficult cases and to provide general assistance, and each major referral hospital should have a lipid clinic.

There is no doubt that if a serious attempt is to be made to reduce the CHD epidemic it is essential that a case-finding approach should be implemented jointly with a strategy aimed at the population as a whole.

Evidence for benefit from an overall approach

In recent years mortality from CHD has fallen considerably in a number of countries, most notably the USA, Australia, and Finland, and it is now falling in England and Wales. It is impossible to establish the explanation for these changing trends with certainty, but they have occurred in parallel with a national will to reduce CHD, dietary change designed to lower blood lipids, a reduction in cigarette smoking, and, perhaps, an increase in physical activity. In Finland, CHD has shown a greater fall in North Karelia than in the rest of Finland (Fig. 11.4). The North Karelia province originally had among the highest CHD rates in Finland and a special CHD intervention project was introduced. It was

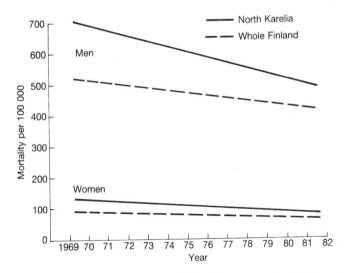

Fig. 11.4 Reduction in CHD in North Karelia compared with the rest of Finland. (Tuomilhelto, J. *et al.* (1986). *British Medical Journal*, **293**, 1068–77.)

originally intended to have an adjacent province as a control group, but it was impossible to prevent lifestyle changes in other provinces in a country so aware of its high CHD risk.

These trends do not provide absolute proof of benefit for a particular lifestyle change, but it is encouraging that the reduction of CHD has been particularly obvious in many countries and communities where special efforts have been made.

Summary

Implementation of the population strategy for CHD prevention is likely to reduce the proportion of people in the population at moderate and high risk. Nevertheless, even with the widespread implementation of dietary advice aimed at reducing population cholesterol concentrations an appreciable proportion will remain at risk. This group will include those with familial hyperlipidaemias and others whose hyperlipidaemia responds inadequately to simple dietary advice. Such people will only be substantially helped by the high-risk approach. A high-risk approach should involve the screening of all those with a family history of CHD or hyperlipidaemia, appreciable obesity, clinical stigmata of hyper-lipidaemia, or any other risk factors for CHD, and ideally doctors should be educated to look for lipid deposits as part of any physical examination.

Extension to offering opportunistic screening to everyone attending the general practitioner's surgery, regardless of the purpose of the visit, would greatly improve the identification of people with hyper-lipidaemia.

12

Screening in primary care

In order to justify the case for screening, certain criteria must be considered. Probably the most important of these is that the disorder is of considerable severity and that effective treatment is available for those detected. Most people consider that these criteria are met for CHD, and that the detection of risk factors is warranted. This would seem particularly true for the inherited conditions such as familial hypercholesterolaemia where the risks of CHD are so high (Fig. 12.1).

A rough estimate of the potential findings in a practice of 10 000 are as follows:

- familial hypercholesterolaemia   20
- other familial hyperlipidaemias   25
- plasma cholesterol >7.5 mmol/l   200
- hypertension (patients under 65)   200

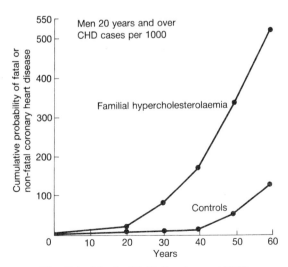

Fig. 12.1 Inherited lipid disorders and CHD.

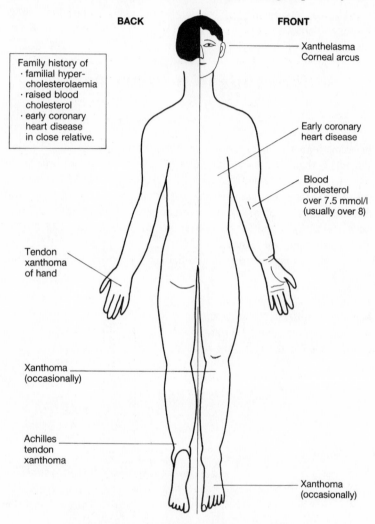

BACK   FRONT

Xanthelasma
Corneal arcus

Family history of
· familial hyper-
  cholesterolaemia
· raised blood
  cholesterol
· early coronary
  heart disease
  in close relative.

Early coronary
heart disease

Blood
cholesterol
over 7.5 mmol/l
(usually over 8)

Tendon
xanthoma
of hand

Xanthoma
(occasionally)

Achilles
tendon
xanthoma

Xanthoma
(occasionally)

Fig. 12.2 Features of familial hypercholesterolaemia.

Screening for cholesterol needs to be part of a general assessment of CHD risk factors. The effect of multiple risk factors on the frequency of CHD is greater than the sum of the individual risk factors (see Fig. 12.3). Even when one risk factor is present to a marked degree, co-incidence of other factors still increases risk.

Table 12.1   Percentage of cases of heterozygous familial
hypercholesterolaemia showing symptoms of CHD,
myocardial infarction (MI), or dying of CHD by age and sex.
(From Goldstein and Brown, 1983; Slack 1969) giving an idea
of the severity of the problem. (Note—many untreated.)

Age to (years)	Males			Females		
	CHD symptoms	MI	CHD death	CHD symptoms	MI	CHD death
30		5%	—	3%	—	—
40	20%		—			
50	45%	51%	25%	20%	12%	2%
60	75%	85%	50%	45%	51%	15%

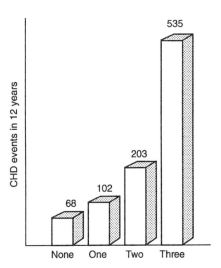

Number of risk factors (serum cholesterol
> 6.5 mmol/l, hypertension, cigarette smoking)

Fig. 12.3   Data from the Framingham study confirm that CHD rises very
steeply when more than one risk factor is present (after Kannel, *Am. J. Cardiol.*
1988). The frequency of cardiac events is almost eight times greater when three
risk factors are present.

The practicalities of organizing screening will vary considerably and the incentives differ between countries and at different times according to government policies. However, a few general considerations and points about the process are made below.

Assessment of problem and overall plan

Decisions need to be made about:

(1) who one intends to screen—sex, age, conditions;
(2) how often one will screen;
(3) which factors one is going to screen for;
(4) how the process is going to be arranged—with regard to organization, patient contact, record keeping, and so on.

Initial assessment:

● *Question about*—symptoms or history of CHD; smoking, alcohol, diet; family history of CHD, especially premature CHD.
● *Look for*—tendon xanthomas/xanthelasma/early corneal arcus.
● *Measure*—weight; blood pressure; random plasma cholesterol; consider fasting cholesterol plus triglycerides if personal or family history of premature CHD, xanthomas present, or if patient has hypertension, diabetes or obesity.
● *Record*—flag notes of patients who are hypertensive, diabetic, hyperlipidaemic, and possibly smokers for follow-up.

For patients found to have a problem, negotiation with the patient is needed to explain the problem, set objectives, and outline time limits in which to achieve these objectives. As some people will have beliefs about their health which will be totally contrary to the advice being given, these beliefs and motivations must be explored and reasons for lifestyle changes found in the group before a major reduction in CHD mortality can be achieved. The plan of follow-up should then be recorded.

Follow-up is required to assess the degree of risk-factor reduction, to update advice, and to ensure that any improvement is maintained. Effective record-keeping is needed. If possible a procedure should be organized to recall defaulters, and to facilitate appropriate rescreening in later years.

Resource requirements

Each practice has to decide what form screening will take after considering the interests and skills of the doctors and nurses in the practice.

Organization of screening on any scale requires energy and time to plan and to monitor, and staff prepared to perform the day-to-day work.

The following priority system for screening has been suggested if resources are limited.

First priority
- patients with known CHD or peripheral vascular disease, especially those who have undergone bypass grafting or other revascularization procedures.
- patients known to have diabetes mellitus or hypertension
- patients with a family history of early CHD
- patients with evident or suspect physical signs suggesting hyperlipidaemia: corneal arcus, xanthelasmas, and xanthomas

Second priority
- patients requesting risk assessment (they are likely to be highly motivated)
- patients in whom brief questioning elicits a family history of CHD presenting before the age of 60 years
- patients who are obviously overweight

Third priority
- other adults

Monitoring the effectiveness of screening

It is not sufficient just to identify CHD risk factors and give advice on lifestyle changes. Staff need to know that as a result the patients do give up smoking, or take exercise and change their diet. Some patients will not understand the message, or not get around to doing anything about it.

Table 12.2 Possible action plan for screening

Smoker	— Counsel on adverse effects Give advice on ceasing; refer to quit smoking programme	Follow-up if possible
Family history of CHD	— Check fasting lipids	
Obese	— Check BP, plasma lipids Advise diet, arrange dietitian visits if appropriate Suggest joining slimming club	Follow-up (nurse/dietitian)
No exercise	— Suggest increase in regular exercise if no contraindications Encourage walking, swimming, etc.	
Hypertension	— BP diastolic 90 mmHg or less — Diastolic >90–114 mmHg — Diastolic 115 mmHg or systolic >160 mmHg Check U & E, urine protein, retina; ECG Diet if obese; stress reduction Arrange for further visits Consider drug treatment if remains elevated	Check in 5 years Check a few weeks later Refer to doctor Regular follow-up
Diabetic	— Check BP, lipids, renal function, proteinuria, eyes, feet, method of glucose monitoring	Regular follow-up
Plasma lipids	— If raised consider: Weight reduction Exclusion of secondary hyperlipidaemia Diet Refer to doctor and consideration of drug treatment if levels remain high on appropriate diet Screen family if index patient appears to have a familial hyperlipidaemia Consider referral to lipid clinic if marked problem	Follow-up of response

How effective is this screening strategy?

Modification of CHD risk factors reduces the incidence of CHD events. The Oslo Heart Study (Chapter 4) demonstrated that individual advice concerning dietary modification and smoking cessation given to a relatively high-risk group of middle-aged men produced major reductions in cholesterol levels and smoking rates. This resulted in a large reduction in CHD events. The STARS and the Lifestyle Heart Study also demonstrated that in people with symptomatic CHD, major reductions in CHD risk factors and arrested progression of coronary atherosclerosis were obtainable by extensive dietary and other lifestyle modifications.

However, two UK studies published in 1994 (*BMJ* **308**:308–12 and 313–18) demonstrated that CHD risk factor screening and modification advice given in general practice to the general UK population produced relatively small overall rates of change in CHD risk factors. The smokers in these studies were low attenders at follow-up, and there was a suggestion that those with 'normal' cholesterol levels reacted by believing that no changes were necessary. Responses may differ in other countries, and need assessment. Prevention programmes must address not only the assessment of CHD risk factors in the individual subjects, but also the meaning and importance of the risk of CHD to them. Someone with symptoms of CHD or a family history of early CHD is likely to feel immediately threatened, and thus strongly motivated to make the necessary changes; whereas someone without symptoms may be unconcerned and resent being made to feel 'unhealthy'.

In the future, research and training must be directed towards improving the skills of those giving advice in primary care. The skills needed include: counselling; understanding the viewpoint of the person receiving the advice; explaining and selling the need to make changes; accurate knowledge of the lifestyle changes needed and their rationales; and plenty of practical guidelines as to how to achieve the changes (what meals to eat, how to buy and prepare them, and whether they fit the person's lifestyle).

Section IV

13

Practical help

The FHA

Several years ago, a number of patients with familial hypercholesterol-aemia (FH) in Britain became very aware of the lack of information generally available. These individuals, assisted by some of their consultants, approached the Simon Broome Heart Research Trust. A self-help group, the Family Heart Association, was thus formed. The aims of the association were:

1. To make the public and the medical profession more aware of this important and fairly common condition.
2. To inform and support those found to have FH.
3. To encourage further research into the cause and treatment of the condition.

The FHA have produced several booklets for patients and for general practitioners and have counsellors who can provide advice and support. The association encourages all people with lipid disorders to join, and receive and contribute suggestions, recipes, which are circulated in a newsletter. An Australian organization was set up in 1988. The remit of the organization has now widened considerably.

The FHA can act as a resource for general practitioners as they have built up contacts with interested GPs, lipid clinic staff, and groups involved with CHD prevention and care.

The following is an example of a booklet to provide an idea of helpful information.

Understanding FH

What is familial hypercholesterolaemia?

Hypercholesterolaemia is the medical name given to the condition of high blood cholesterol. 'Hyper' means raised; Cholesterol is the fatty substance described below, and 'aemia' means in the blood. People with high blood cholesterol tend to have a greater risk of developing coronary heart disease.

Familial hypercholesterolaemia (FH)

Is the name given to high blood cholesterol where it is inherited and passed from parent to child.

What is cholesterol?

Cholesterol is one of the fatty substances present in the blood and all body tissues. It is an important part of the outer envelopes of each cell in the body. Cholesterol comes partly from the diet, and is also made by the body.

What is high blood cholesterol?

People with high blood cholesterol have an amount of cholesterol in their blood which is higher than normal for people in this country.

The body normally maintains a delicate balance between the cholesterol eaten, the cholesterol made in the liver, and the amount required by the body so that supply matches demand. In FH there is an inherited abnormality in the cells of the body which upsets this balance so that the level of cholesterol in the blood is high and there is a gradual build-up of fatty cholesterol deposits in the body.

People with high blood cholesterol tend to have a greater risk of developing coronary heart disease.

What is coronary heart disease?

Coronary heart disease is the name given to the narrowing of the coronary arteries which convey blood to the heart. The narrowing is caused by a build-up of fatty cholesterol deposits which, in time, could severely restrict the amount of blood reaching the heart. If this happens suddenly there may be damage to part of the heart muscle—this is known as a heart attack (coronary thrombosis). With FH this can happen in relatively young people.

Statistics show that men run a greater risk of developing coronary heart disease than women. There are also other factors apart from high blood cholesterol that increase the risk of developing heart disease. These include smoking, lack of exercise, overeating leading to obesity, diabetes, and high blood pressure.

Diagnosing FH

How can you tell if you have FH?

If members of your family, whether one of your parents, uncles, aunts, brothers, or sisters, has had a heart attack (coronary thrombosis) at a young age—in early or middle adult life—this could be because of FH. Other indications of the conditions are:

1. Xanthomas—these are swellings in the tendons on the back of the hands or ankles as a result of a build-up of cholesterol here.
2. Corneal arcus—a white band towards the end of the coloured part of the eye in younger people (under 50 years). The band may occur without FH, and indeed without any change in cholesterol, in older people.
3. Xanthelasmas—yellow lumps or streaks of fat in the skin close to the eye.
4. High blood cholesterol in a close relative.

If any of these apply to you, you should first consult your family doctor and have your blood cholesterol and other fats measured.

The outward signs of FH are not present in all patients, and even when they are they may cause little or no discomfort or inconvenience. However, they do help the doctor in making the diagnosis.

Not everyone with high blood cholesterol has FH, but it makes a good deal of sense to have the tests.

If someone in your family is known to have FH then IT IS VERY IMPORTANT that all members of the family ask their doctor to check their blood cholesterol.

Can FH miss a generation then reappear in grandchildren?

FH does not miss a generation, but because it does not always result in a heart attack at an early age, it may sometimes not be diagnosed if the blood cholesterol is not measured.

Reducing the risk

Can the risk of heart attacks be removed or reduced if blood cholesterol can be lowered?

High blood cholesteriol increases the risk. Lowering blood cholesterol is the essential basis for treatment. Once FH is diagnosed, treatment should be started as soon as possible, before disease has developed in the coronary arteries.

Diet is a very important factor in lowering cholesterol levels in the blood.

Must I always keep to my diet?

Departures from the diet on special occasions will not cause problems, provided you normally keep carefully to your diet. It is the average diet over a period of time that is important. Remember, though, that there is a danger of finding too many excuses for special occasions!

How can I make my children's diet more interesting?

It is difficult for children to keep to a special diet which excludes chocolate, cakes, and crisps among other things. The following tips may help.

Sandwiches can be made with tuna and cucumber, chicken, lean roast beef and ham, cottage cheese, and other low-fat cheeses, with tomato, pickle, pineapple, yeast extract, jam, and honey. You can also pack individual salads in a plastic container. Add a piece of fruit, carton of yoghurt, muesli biscuits, slice of bran and banana loaf or some dried fruit.

Encourage your children to eat more vegetables. Try cooking the vegetables in different ways. Make the children 'polyunsaturated' crisps. Using a potato peeler, cut slices very finely, rinse under the tap, pat dry, and deep fry in polyunsaturated oil. These are much cheaper than commercially bought ones.

What about my weight?

People with FH should try to avoid being overweight because it is more difficult to keep blood cholesterol down. Also being overweight itself increases the risk of developing heart disease.

What about alcohol?

Yes, it is fine to have a social drink, but remember, if you have a weight problem, that it is fattening.

Should I continue to smoke?

NO, smoking is a disaster! Smoking is already associated with a high risk of heart attacks so it is particularly dangerous when FH has been diagnosed.

Is it safe to take exercise—or ever play sports?

An active lifestyle, including pursuits such as walking, cycling, swimming, and gardening, is to be encouraged in helping to prevent coronary heart disease. However, if you have not previously been active you should take up exercise very gradually. In adults with FH who may have some narrowing of the coronary arteries without symptoms of heart disease, sudden vigorous exertion and high competitive physical sports are probably best avoided. Discuss your exercise plans with your doctor.

Information for doctors and patients

Other booklets on CHD risk factors are available from the Heart Foundations and other organisations such as The British Heart Foundation, 102 Gloucester Place, London W1, The National Heart Foundation of Australia—which has offices in a number of cities (head office in Canberra), and the National Heart Foundation of New Zealand PO Box 17160, Greenlane, Auckland 5. Up-to-date readable reviews on lipid topics can be found in Lipid Reviews, which is published by Current Medical Literature Ltd, 40 Osnaburgh Street, London NW1. Current opinions in Lipidology provides a more comprehensive review of topics of interests.

Public awareness

Community attitudes to people who wish to lead a different lifestyle from the generally accepted norm can be hostile. This can apply to people who wish to change their lifestyle because of hyperlipidaemia. Individuals may find resentment to their requests for 'low-fat' foods in work canteens, and parents often complain that they have difficulty over school meals for their children. Hopefully, campaigns aimed at canteens, such as the NZ Heartbeat award, may improve the knowledge of some caterers.

Health professionals and the public need more education about the importance of hyperlipidaemia and other CHD risk factors, and their treatment. In this way a gradual change in attitudes can hopefully be achieved. The food industry in general, both manufacturers and retailers, have shown little concern about the need for a prudent diet which would reduce the risk of CHD for the whole population, as well as special high-risk groups. The food chain is complex and includes producers, processors, manufacturers, distributers, caterers, government departments, and the consumer. Complicated and sometimes conflicting interests are involved. Changes are really needed in agricultural policies, for example, to encourage farmers to produce leaner meat and to increase the production of cereals, vegetables, and fruit. This would of course have far reaching implications.

The situation is improving slowly. Information on diet and CHD is now quite widely available, and some school courses are including more information on nutrition. Much still remains to be done, however, particularly within certain social groups. Some food manufacturers are realizing that there is a growing market for 'health-promoting' foods. Several supermarket chains now stock low-fat, high-fibre foods which are well labelled, and provide leaflets and information on healthy eating. Alternatives of packaged or tinned food are available without added sugar, salt, and preservatives, in some shops. The information on processed foods is generally improving, but there is still a long way to go. Food labelling needs to be dramatically improved to include the fat content, its source, and the percentage of saturated and unsaturated fat, as well as other nutritional information. Initiatives in several countries are aimed at providing simple markers for consumers to identify healthy food options, such as the 'tick' system endorsed by The Australian Heart Foundation and although these may have their problems they are very helpful to some consumers.

RECIPES

The following section includes a selection of recipes for low-fat meals.

Main courses

1   Chicken, ham, and apple salad

Serves 4
Each serving: 210 kcal, 10 g fibre, 4 g fat

2 medium-sized apples (red or green, cored, and diced)
100 g (3½ oz) cooked chicken or turkey, diced
100 g (3½ oz) cooked lean ham, diced
200 g (7 oz) cooked peas
3 large stalks of celery, chopped
30 g (1 oz sultanas)
Lettuce

Mix ingredient except lettuce—lay on bed of lettuce. Use 50 ml (¼ pint) of low-fat plain yoghurt plus seasoning as dressing.
Serve with cooked brown rice (½ cup per person) mixed with sweetcorn kernels.

2   Country vegetable risotto

Serves 4
Each serving: 440 kcal, 23 g fibre, 1 g fat

200 g (7 oz) haricot beans or kidney beans
1 tbsp polyunsaturated oil
1 medium-size onion, chopped
1 clove garlic (optional)
3 large carrots, diced
⅓ tsp salt and pepper
1 tbsp marjoram or sage

400 ml (14 fl oz) stock
200 g (7 oz) long-grain brown rice
200 g (7 oz) fresh or frozen peas
3 tbsp chopped parsley
1 bunch spring onions, green and white parts, sliced
30 g (1 oz) parmesan cheese

Cook the beans or use drained tinned beans. Heat the oil in a saucepan and fry the onion and garlic for a few minutes. Add the carrots and swede and continue to cook, stirring occasionally, for 3–4 minutes. Sprinkle the seasoning and marjoram or sage into the pan, cover with water and simmer for 20–25 minutes, or until almost tender. Drain.

Meanwhile, in another saucepan, bring the stock to the boil, sprinkle in the rice, stir, and return to the boil. Lower the heat, cover the pan, and cook gently for 30–35 minutes, adding more stock until the rice is almost tender and the stock absorbed. Add the beans, peas, and the cooked vegetables, and continue cooking for 10 minutes. Remove from the heat, adjust the seasoning, mix in half the parsley, pile onto a hot serving dish, and garnish with the remaining parsley, spring onions, and cheese. The consistency should be moist and creamy.

An alternative method is to boil the beans until half-cooked, then add the vegetables and rice. As different kinds of beans and brown rice vary in the cooking time required, the first method ensures the beans are properly cooked. The alternative cooking method, however, produces a dish with a very low fat content.

Many other vegetables may be used—unpeeled diced potatoes, courgettes, broad beans, green beans, leeks, and so on.

3   White fish in white sauce

White fish (cod, haddock, plaice, coley, whiting, halibut)
2–4 oz per person
Skimmed milk
Potato powder
Parsley or pepper

Thaw fish (if frozen) and place in saucepan, cover with
skimmed milk (about ⅓ pint per person) and bring to the boil.
Simmer for 30 seconds (for plaice) to 2 minutes (cod). Drain
milk into basin and add potato powder until sauce is desired
thickness, stirring continuously. Cover fish with sauce and
sprinkle with parsley. Serve with boiled potatoes and
vegetables of choice.

4 Pasta and meat/vegetable sauce and grated cheese

Pasta 50 g (2 oz) per person: spaghetti, pasta whirls, or
macaroni (preferably high fibre or wholemeal)
Small amount of diced ham, low-fat mince, diced chicken, or
turkey.
Onion, peppers, mushrooms, courgettes, kidney beans, chick
peas, or other similar pulses
Tin of tomatoes

Cook pasta according to packet instructions.
Fry vegetables in a small amount of polyunsaturated
margarine.
Add tomatoes and simmer for 5 minutes
Drain pasta, pour sauce over pasta. Sprinkle with grated or
parmesan cheese and black pepper.

5 Chicken lasagne

Serves 4
Each serving: 380 kcal, 40 g (4 units) carbohydrate, 9 g fibre,
26 g protein, 13 g fat.

140 g (5 oz) wholemeal lasagne
15 ml (1 tbsp) corn oil
1 large onion, chopped
1 clove garlic, crushed
400 g (14 oz) tomatoes
1½ tbsp marjoram
4 outer stalks celery, diced and lightly cooked
6 tbsp chopped green pepper

170 g (6 oz) chopped chicken, diced
seasoning
30 g (1 oz) cheese, grated
Sauce:
1 small onion, chopped
Carrot, chopped
Turnip, chopped
425 ml (¾ pint) skimmed milk
30 g (3 tbsp) wholemeal flour
15 g (½ oz) polyunsaturated margarine
Seasoning

Garnish: paprika

Heat the oven to 190 °C/374 °F/gas 5.
Cook the lasagne in boiling salted water until half-cooked,
drain carefully. Heat the oil and cook the onion and garlic for
5 minutes, until soft. Add the tomatoes, marjoram, celery,
peppers, chicken, and seasoning, and cook for 5 minutes. To
make the sauce, simmer the vegetables, bay leaf, and mace in
nearly all the milk for 15 minutes. Remove the bay leaf and
mace and mix the ingredients in a blender. Return to the pan
and bring to the boil.

Meanwhile, blend the flour with the remaining milk. Stir
the hot milk into the flour, add the margarine and seasonings,
return to pan and cook gently for a few minutes. Place the
chicken mixture, sauce, and lasagne in alternate layers in a
dish, finishing with sauce. Scatter the cheese evenly over the
top and cook for 30–35 minutes. Sprinkle a little paprika on
top and serve.

This dish can be prepared in advance to this stage, cooked,
covered and stored in the refrigerator, but allow 40–45
minutes for the final cooking.

6   Chilli con carne

Serves 4
Each serving: 530 kcal, 60 g (6 units) carbohydrates, 27 g fibre,
37 g protein, 16 g fat.

30 ml (2 tbsp) corn oil or rapeseed oil
2 medium-sized onions, chopped
1 clove garlic, crushed
170 g (6 oz) lean minced meat
20 g (2 tbsp) wholemeal flour
2 tbsp tomato puree
250 ml (9 fl oz) stock, hot
1–3 tsp chilli powder
400 g (14 oz) canned tomatoes
450 g (1 lb) red kidney beans, soaked or canned
salt
1 medium/large green pepper, chopped

Heat the oil and gently fry onions, and garlic for 5 minutes. Toss the meat in flour, add to the onions, and cook until brown, stirring. Mix tomato puree with the hot stock and gradually stir into the meat. Add the chilli powder, tomatoes, and beans, and boil for 10 minutes. Stir, cover tightly, and simmer gently for 1–1¼ hours until the beans are cooked. Ten minutes before serving stir in salt and the green pepper.

Use a mixture of meat and textured vegetable protein, or soya soaked in a small amount of hot water and marmite, in place of all meat. Instead of red kidney beans, use haricot, butter, or soya beans. The cooking time should be adjusted.

7 Vegetarian bean paella

Serves 4
Each serving: 420 kcal, 70 g (7 units) carbohydrate, 20 g fibre, 16 g protein, 10 g fat.

100 g (3½ oz) red kidney beans
60 g (2 oz) mung or haricot beans
225 g (8 oz) long-grain brown rice
450 ml (¾ pint) water
½ tsp turmeric (optional)
1 small aubergine, diced
30 ml (2 tbsp) corn oil
1 onion, chopped
1 stick celery chopped
1 medium large green pepper, chopped

2 large carrots, diced
300 g (10½ oz) canned tomatoes, drained
115 g (4 oz) button mushrooms
Seasoning
2 tbsp chopped parsley
Saffron

Cook the beans. Meanwhile, put the rice, water, saffron and
1 tsp salt in a saucepan and cook for 30 minutes. Sprinkle salt
over the aubergine, leave for 20 minutes, then wipe dry. Heat
the oil in another saucepan and gently cook the onion and
garlic for 5 minutes. Add the aubergine, celery, green pepper,
and carrots and cook gently, stirring occasionally, for 10
minutes. Stir in the tomatoes and mushrooms, and continue
cooking for 5 minutes. Gently mix the vegetables and beans
into the rice, adjust the seasoning if necessary. Cover the pan
and continue cooking gently for 15 minutes. Turn off the heat
and keep the mixture warm for 10 minutes. Gently fork in the
parsley and serve.

Accompaniments

8   Parsley rice

Serves 4
Each serving: 270 kcal, 6 g fibre, 2 g fat.

225 g (8 oz) long-grain brown rice
30 g (1 oz) polyunsaturated margarine
1 large bunch spring onions, sliced
4 stalks of celery
6 tbsp chopped parsley or other fresh herbs
seasoning

Cook the rice. Meanwhile, melt the margarine in a saucepan.
Add the spring onions and celery and fry gently, stirring occasionally, for 7–10 minutes or until just tender. Add the freshly
cooked, moist rice and chopped parsley, adjust the seasoning,
and allow to heat through thoroughly, stirring occasionally.
Serve as an accompaniment to a main course.

9 Mackerel pate
1 tin mackerel 150 g
1 tin butter beans 8 oz
Pepper
Mix mackerel, pepper, and butter beans together. Mash with
fork or in a food processor (if available). Place in serving dish.

Sweets

10   Apple oatmeal crumble

Serves 4–6
Each serving: 230 cal, 40 g (4 units) carbohydrate, 7 g fibre, 7 g
fat.

570 g (1¼ lb) cooking apples, cored
¼–½ tsp ground cloves
Low-calorie or sugar-free sweetener to taste
60 ml (4 tbsp) hot water
30 g (4 tbsp) rolled oats
100 g (3½ oz) wholemeal flour
30 g (1 oz) polyunsaturated margarine

Heat the oven to 180 °C/350 °F/gas 4. Slice the apples in
cross-cut slices to avoid long strips of peel. Place in a baking
dish, sprinkle with the cloves, and add the sweetener to taste.
Mix together the oats and flour, and rub in the margarine.
Sprinkle over the fruit and bake for 30–40 minutes.
Other fruits, such as rhubarb or plums, can be used.

11   Rhubard charlotte

Serves 4
Each serving: 130 cal, 20 g (2 units) carbohydrate, 7 g fibre, 4 g
fat.

450 g (1 lb) young rhubarb*
170 g (6 oz) wholemeal breadcrumbs
grated rind of 1 orange
½ tsp ground ginger

60 ml (4 tbsp) orange juice
¼ tsp ground cinnamon and nutmeg (optional)
low calorie or sugar-free liquid sweetener to taste
30 g (1 oz) low-fat spread

Heat the oven to 190 °C/375°F/gas 5
Cut rhubarb in 2.5 cm (1 inch) lengths and place in a layer in a
non-stick pie dish or casserole. Sprinkle a layer of breadcrumbs on top. Mix together orange rind, ginger, cinnamon,
and nutmeg, if used, and sprinkle a little over the breadcrumbs. Repeat the layers finishing with a layer of breadcrumbs, but before the final layer, pour over the orange juice
mixed with sweetener. Dot the final layer of breadcrumbs with
the low-fat spread. Cover and bake for 10–15 minutes until the
top is crisp and lightly brown. Serve hot.

*Older rhubarb may be used, but stew gently with a litter water to part-cook
before assembling the pudding.

Some of these recipes are adapted from ones given in 'The Healthy Heart Diet
Book' by Longstaff and Mann and the 'Diabetics' Diet Book' by J. Mann,
published by Martin Dunitz.

Recipes using Questran or Questran lite (cholestyramine or colestid)

Soft drinks/Fruit juices

1 sachet of Questran
250 ml (8 fl oz) soft drink any flavour, or fruit juice

Put Questran powder in a large glass. Add 3–4 oz soft drink or
juice and stir until all Questran is in suspension. (This will
cause the soft drink to foam.) Add rest of fluid slowly, and stir
gently. Low-calorie soft drinks should usually be used in
place of sugar-sweetened drinks for adults.

Milk shakes

250 ml (8 fl oz) skimmed milk
2 teaspoons milk-shake powder
1 sachet of Questran

Combine the powders together in a glass. Gradually add the milk, stirring all the time. A liquidized banana can be used instead of milk-shake powder.

Yoghurt drink

150 g (5 oz) raspberry yoghurt or any low-fat fruit-flavoured yoghurt
125 ml (¼ pint) skimmed milk
1 sachet of Questran

Mix everything together and stir thoroughly until evenly dispersed.

Hot lemon

Use lemon juice or lemon squash or other fruit cordial.
First add hot water to make one cup, then add one Questran sachet and stir thoroughly until Questran is in suspension.

Ginger special

10 ml (4 fl oz) orange juice or lime juice
250 ml (8 fl oz) ginger ale or low-calorie ginger ale
2 sachets of Questran
Ice cubes if required

Sprinkle Questran into orange juice and stir thoroughly until Questran is evenly dispersed. Add ginger ale. Stir.

Porridge

Porridge oats (quantity as recommended by manufacturer)
Skimmed milk
1 sachet Questran

Prepare porridge according to package directions using skimmed milk and 1/4 cup more water than directions suggest. When cooked remove from heat and sprinkle one sachet of Questran into an individual portion and mix thoroughly. If porridge is too thick, stir in more hot water.

Caribbean yoghurt breakfast

2 × 5 oz (150 g) cartons of low-fat natural or fruit yoghurt
1–2 tsp muscovado sugar (if required)
1 pinch cinnamon
1 tbsp sultanas
1 grapefruit (segmented)
1 tbsp of muesli
1 sachet Questran

Mix all ingredients except Questran. Divide into two servings and add Questran to individual portion, stir thoroughly. This recipe can be used with many other fruits—fresh orange, apple, melon, banana, or pineapple.

Chicken/turkey casserole

Serves 4

10 oz uncooked chicken or turkey (without skin)
14 oz mixed vegetables, carrots/sweetcorn/beans/peas/celery
1¾ pints boiling chicken stock
Black pepper/soy sauce seasoning

Mix ingredients and cook for 1½ hours. Dissolve Questran in small amount of warm water and mix in thoroughly with portion.

Some of these recipes are adapted from ones given in a booklet produced by Bristol Myers.

Eating out, packed snacks, and buffet meals

Eating out

If possible choose somewhere to eat where you know the menu will include simply cooked food rather than elaborate made-up dishes with unknown ingredients. Contact a number of restaurants in advance to find whether they have suitable meals.

Starters
Fruit, fruit juice, tomato juice.
Avoid pate, cream soup, shellfish cocktail.

Main course
Fish; grilled or poached.
Poultry, roast or grilled meat, cold meat: trim off any obvious fat or skin.
Avoid sauces, stuffings, dumplings, pastry.

Vegetables
All salads, add dressing of oil and vinegar at the table.
Any vegetable prepared without fat or sauce.
Jacket or boiled potatoes
Avoid salads, already mixed together with rich creamy dressings, and creamed, roast, or fried vegetables.

Bread
Wholemeal bread or rolls, crispbreads.
Avoid butter.

Dessert
Fresh or canned fruit, jelly, sorbet.
Avoid cream, rich creamy ice creams, pies, and gateaux.

To drink
Fruit juice, mineral water, or moderate amounts of wine, beer and spirit (if permitted). Coffee, tea.
Avoid cream in coffee or tea.

Remember If it is impossible to avoid some unsuitable food, have a small helping and satisfy your appetite with generous helpings of other foods. The occasional small lapse will not cause harm, but it is important to return immediately to your recommended dietary routine.

Packed snacks

It is probably sensible to try to find suitable containers for certain foods.

Soups
Main course or light soups (low-calorie or home-made with low-fat content) carried in a thermos flask on cold days.

Wholemeal rolls or sandwiches (in plastic snap bags) or crispbreads.
Spread sparingly with mono- or polyunsaturated margarine, low-fat margarine or cheese spreads, or low-calorie salad dressings. Alternatively, just use a filling made very moist and tasty.

Fillings can include: slices of poultry, lean meat or ham—or mince these and mix with chutney, pickles, or low-fat sauce; canned fish mixed with vinegar, low-fat salad dressing, tomato puree, or bottled sauce; cottage or low-fat curd cheese mixed with herbs, sauce, pickles, chopped salad vegetables, or chopped grapes; home-made pate spread directly on to bread.

To the above fillings, add sliced or shredded salad ingredients and home-made salad dressings, or have carrots/celery/tomatoes separately.

In cartons
Salads of vegetables, brown rice, and pasta mixed with chopped poultry, lean ham, or fish, and permitted salad dressings.

Dessert
Fresh or dried fruit and nuts.
Cold desserts in seal-top containers. Low-fat yoghurt.
Biscuits baked with appropriate ingredients.

To drink
Cold drinks in seal-top tumblers. Coffee or tea with skimmed milk.
Sometimes: canned beer, bottle or cartons of wine, or non-alcoholic wine.

Catering for buffet meals

Select from the following foods:

Starters
Melon, grapefruit, fruit juice.
Home-made pate (see recipes) with wholemeal melba toast.
Mixed vegetable broth with added wholemeal cereals, pulse soups, and croutons of wholemeal bread, toasted or fried in polyunsaturated oil.

Main courses
Moderate amounts of fish, meat, and cheese extended by combining with wholemeat cereals and vegetables, and presented to make a variety of dishes. For example, flans, pizzas, risottos, pasta with succulent meat or fish sauces, casseroles with pulses and other vegetables, salmon (or other fish) mousse.

Vegetables
Colourful salads made from summer and winter vegetables combined with pulses, brown rice, and pastas.
Crisply cooked vegetables.
Rice/sweetcorn/pepper mixes.
Potatoes baked or boiled in skins with low-fat cheese or dressing.

Dressings
Home-made French or yoghurt dressings.
Proprietary low-calorie dressings.
Olive oil.

Bread
Wholemeal wheat bread, rye bread, and rolls, crispbreads, oatcakes.
French bread sticks warmed in the oven.

Spreads
Tubs of mono-or polyunsaturated margarine, low-fat margarine spread and home-made, low-calorie spreads. Some polyunsaturated margarines and spreads may be made into 'pats' using a butter curler.

Desserts
Fresh fruit.

Fresh fruit made up into fruit jellies and flans.
Fruity puddings such as charlottes and pies made with appropriate thin
pastry (polyunsaturated fat and half brown/half white flour).
Sorbets, home-made ice cream.

Information sheet for patients on dietary principles

*What part does diet play in the treatment of hyperlipidaemia
(high blood fats)?*

Dietary modification is the first line of treatment in hyperlipidaemia.
The ideal diet is one which aims to achieve ideal body weight, is low in
fat, and has a relatively high ratio of mono- and polyunsaturated fat to
saturated fat, and a high content of dietary fibre. In the typical affluent
Western diet, about 36–40 per cent of all calories come from fat, 45 per
cent from carbohydrate, and 15 per cent from protein. For those with
hyperlipidaemia, fat should be reduced to less than 30 per cent of total
calories. This should be done by decreasing saturated fat. Fibre-rich
carbohydrate should be increased. This way of eating has been
endorsed by official recommendations throughout the world as a major
way of reducing the epidemic of coronary heart disease. It is suitable
for the whole family whether or not they have hyperlipidaemia. Those
who do not have raised lipid levels can be less strict.

Important points about your diet

These general guidelines will help you to follow a healthy balanced
eating pattern. The same dietary principles apply to all types of hyperlipidaemia, though some aspects may be particularly emphasized for
people with certain conditions.

Eat less fat.   It is important to eat less fat as the amounts you eat will
influence cholesterol levels in your blood. Note that *all fats* are high in
calories. Avoid fried and fatty foods (remember there are hidden fats in
many foods, such as meats, dairy products, nuts, cakes, biscuits, choco-
lates). Be sparing with all cooking and spreading fats and use products
with mono- or polyunsaturated fats. Wherever possible, choose low-fat
alternatives of foods.

Practical help

Use monounsaturated or polyunsaturated fats in preference to saturated fats. The type of fat you choose in your diet will affect the level of cholesterol in your blood. Saturated fats (mainly from dairy and animal sources) tend to raise blood cholesterol while mono- and polyunsaturated fats (from some vegetable and fish oils) can help to lower it. Therefore, it is beneficial to choose monounsaturated fats (for example, olive or rapeseed oil) and polyunsaturated fats (such as sunflower, corn, or soya oil/margarine) in preference to saturated types (for example, butter, margarine, lard, or dripping).

NB Not all vegetable fats are polyunsaturated. Choose vegetable oil or margarine labelled high in mono- or polyunsaturates.

Eat more fibre-containing foods. A high-fibre diet is known to be beneficial to health. Some types of fibre commonly called soluble fibre, are especially useful in helping to lower blood cholesterol. These are found in legumes and pulses (dried peas, beans, and lentils), as pectins in fruits, and in porridge oats and oatmeal. Ensure you have plenty of fibre in your diet by including wholegrain cereals, wholemeal bread, plenty of vegetables and fruit, and regularly use pulses such as haricot beans, red kidney beans, and butter beans to name but a few of the very wide range available.

Cholesterol. While it is important not to take excessive amounts of cholesterol in food, it is far more important to watch the fat content of your diet. Eating too much saturated fat will cause far more harm than a small intake of cholesterol-rich foods. Therefore, it is more essential to take an overall low-fat diet than simply a low-cholesterol diet.

Sugar. Some foods which are high in fat (such as chocolate, biscuits, cakes, puddings, sweet pastries) also contain sugar and are high in calories. These should be avoided. Other sugary foods (for example, jam, marmalade, honey) need to be reduced if you are trying to lose weight or if triglycerides are raised.

Alcohol. All forms of alcohol are high in calories and should be restricted if you are overweight. In addition, there is some evidence that alcohol may raise triglyceride levels. No one should drink excessively, but some people with hyperlipidaemia, specifically raised triglycerides, need to restrict alcohol consumption.

Appendix

Lipid metabolism: expanded notes

Apoproteins

These are the lipid-free protein components of the plasma lipoproteins. In general they are involved in maintaining structural integrity of the lipoprotein particles and they have a role in receptor recognition and enzyme regulation. They are classed A, B, C, D, and E with subclasses. Apoprotein A is the major protein in HDL. Apo A1 binds phospholipid, activates lecithin cholesterol acyltransferase, and may have a function in regulation of membrane lipids and membrane fluidity. Apo A11 has a structural function. Apoprotein B constitutes 90 per cent of the protein of LDL and is a major protein of chylomicrons and VLDL. It is thought to have a vital function in the transport of triglycerides. Apoprotein CII activates the lipoprotein lipase of adipose tissue. Apoprotein E is involved with recognition of the remnant particle by the liver. Various isoforms exist and a person's ability to clear remnants rapidly may depend on their apo E phenotype.

Fat absorption

Fats constitute 40 per cent of the calorie intake of many people. Partial hydrolysis of ingested fats occurs in the small intestine, due to the action of lipases, and in the presence of the bile salts, cholic and chenodeoxycholic acid, and some phospholipids, micelles are formed. Monoglycerides and non-esterified fatty acids are absorbed in the duodenum and proximal jejunum, and are re-esterified in the endothelial cells to form triglycerides.

Dietary cholesterol esters are hydrolysed by pancreatic enzymes, and the cholesterol is absorbed in the small intestine. In the intestinal epithelial cells, triglycerides combine with cholesterol, phospholipids and specific apoliproteins which have been absorbed or synthesized by the mucosal cells. The lipoproteins formed (chylomicrons and intestinal VLDL) are rich in triglyceride and are secreted into the lymphatic system where changes in cholesterol, phospholipid, and apoproteins occur, including loss of apo A11 and uptake of apoproteins C and E.

Fat transport

Chylomicrons enter the blood from the lymphatic system and may cause turbidity of the plasma after a fat-rich meal. Because triglycerides are insoluble in plasma they are transported as lipoproteins—macromolecular aggregates of variable size, lipid, and protein content. These lipoproteins are usually classified by density on ultracentrifugation. The lowest density lipoprotein with the greatest triglyceride content has the highest flotation number.

	Lipoprotein flotation (Sf)	Main lipid	Main apoprotein
Chylomicrons	10^3–10^5	triglyceride	B
VLDL (very low density lipoprotein)	20–400	triglyceride	B, C, E
LDL (low density lipoprotein)	0–20	cholesterol	B
HDL (high density lipoprotein)		phospholipid	A, D

VLDL is also synthesized in the liver, and is the transport form of endogenously synthesized triglyceride.

In the circulation, triglyceride is gradually removed from the chylomicrons and VLDL, mainly by the action of lipoprotein lipase. Lipoprotein lipase is present in the capillaries of a number of tissues, but predominantly in adipose tissue and skeletal muscle, and it is stimulated by apoprotein CII present in the triglyceride-rich lipoprotein particles. Lipoprotein lipase is also stimulated by insulin and reduced activity occurs in poorly controlled diabetes.

Glycerides and non-esterified fatty acids removed largely by lipase action are taken up by muscle or adipose cells. These fatty acids provide the main energy source for aerobic metabolism in muscle and in a well-fed individual the excess is stored as triglyceride. As the triglycerides are removed the remnant particle becomes smaller and some of the more water soluble components on the surface become redundant. These include phospholipid, unesterified cholesterol, and the apo C molecules, which transfer to HDL. Cholesterol ester transfer protein appears to facilitate this transfer of cholesterol esters to HDL, and the passage of some triglycerides from HDL to VLDL. The metabolism of the chylomicron remnant or IDL is controversial. Some is probably taken up by the liver, and some is metabolized in the plasma to LDL. LDL is rich in cholesterol. Removal of LDL from the circulation is slower than that of many other particles. About half the LDL is initially bound by high-affinity cell receptors, and apoproteins B and E in the particle probably aid this binding. LDL then enters the cell and is degraded in lysosomes to liberate cholesterol which can be used by the cell. Dietary cholesterol inhibits endogenous cholesterol synthesis by inhibiting an enzyme in the pathway of cholesterol synthesis. The number of cell receptors appears to be regulated by the intracellular cholesterol level. There is also a low-affinity receptor pathway, which is not known to be regulated, but which becomes proportionally more important at higher LDL concentration. The activity of the high-affinity receptor is a major determinant of plasma LDL and cholesterol levels, and disorders affecting these receptors, such as occur in familial hypercholesterolaemia, have marked effects upon cholesterol metabolism and circulating plasma levels.

The other group of lipoproteins in the circulation are HDL_1, HDL_2 and HDL_3. These are mainly synthesized in the intestinal mucosa and liver. Phospholipids and cholesterol which become redundant when triglyceride-rich lipoproteins are metabolized are transferred to these particles, particularly the small HDL_3 particle which becomes transformed into the larger HDL_2 particle and where cholesterol esters are formed by the action of lecithin cholesterol acyl transferase. These cholesterol esters may then transfer to other particles. The particular interest in this lipoprotein has arisen because the level of HDL_2 is inversely related to the risk of CHD.

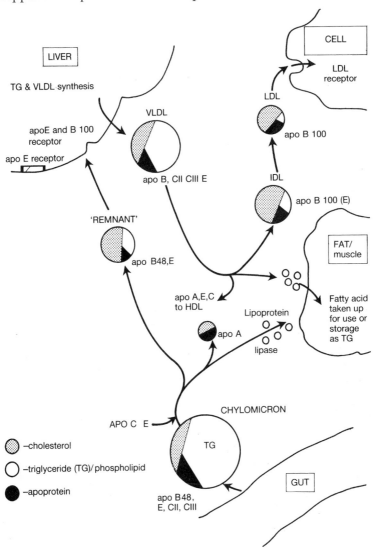

Fig. A.1 Pictorial summary of lipoprotein metabolism.

References and further reading

Epidemiological studies

Castelli, W.P. (1986). The triglyceride issue: A view from Framingham. *Am. Heart J.*, **112**, 432–7.

Gey, K. *et al.* (1991). Inverse correlation between plasma vitamin E and mortality from ischemic heart disease in cross-cultural epidemiology. *Am. J. Clin. Nutr*, **53**, S326–45.

Gouldbourt, U., Holtzman, E., and Neufeld, H.N. (1985). Total and high density lipoprotein cholesterol in the serum and risk of mortality: evidence of a threshold effect. *Br. Med. J.*, **290**, 1239–43.

Gordon, T., Kannel, W.B., Castelli, W.B., and Dawber, T.R. (1981). Lipoproteins, cardiovascular disease and death. The Framingham study. *Arch. Intern. Med.*, **141**, 1128–31.

Life in New Zealand Survey. (1991). Otago University.

Meade, T., Mellow, S., Brozovic, M., *et al.* (1986). Haemostatic function and ischaemic heart disease: principal results of the Northwick Park Heart Study. *Lancet*, **2**, 533–7.

National Heart Foundation of Australia. (1989). Risk factor prevalence study. *Survey No. 3.*

Pekkanen, J. *et al.* (1990). Ten-year mortality from cardiovascular disease in relation to cholesterol level among men with and without pre-existing cardiovascular disease. *New Engl. J. Med.*, **322**, 1700–7.

Pocock, S.J., Shaper, A.G., Phillips, A.N., Walker, M., and Whitehead, T.P. (1986). High density lipoprotein cholesterol is not a major risk factor for ischaemic heart disease in British men. *Br. Med. J.*, **292**, 515–19.

Stone, N.J., Levy, R.I., Fredrickson, D.S., and Verter, J. (1974). Coronary artery disease in 116 kindred with familial type II hyperlipoproteinemia. *Circulation*, **49**, 476–80.

Diet

Berry, E. *et al.* (1991). Effects of diets rich in mono-unsaturated fatty acids on plasma lipoproteins. *Am. J. Clin. Nutr.* **53**, 899–907.

Department of Health (1991). *Dietary reference values for food energy and nutrients for the United Kingdom.* Report 41. HMSO, London.

Edington, J., Geekie, M., Carter, R., Benfield, L., Fisher, K., Ball, M., and Mann, J. (1987). Effect of dietary cholesterol on plasma cholesterol concentration in subjects following reduced fat, high fibre diet. *Br. Med. J.*, **294**, 333–6.

Food for Health. (1991). *The Report of the Nutrition Task Force to the Department of Health.* Department of Health, Wellington, New Zealand. ISBN 0-477-07538-X.

Garg, A. and Grundy, S. (1990). Management of dyslipidaemia in NIDDM. *Diabetes Care*, **13**, 153–64.

Grundy, S.M. and Denke, M.A. (1990). Dietary influences on serum lipids and lipoproteins. *J. Lipid Res.*, **31**, 1149–72.

Herold, P. and Kinsella, J. (1986). Fish oil consumption and decreased risk of cardiovascular disease: comparison of findings from animal and human feeding trials. *Am. J. Clin. Nutr.*, **43**, 566–98.

Keys, A., Anderson, J.T., and Grande, F. (1965). Serum cholesterol response to changes in diet. II. The effect of cholesterol in the diet. *Metabolism*, **14**, 759–65.

Mann, J. and the Oxford Dietetic Group. (1982). *The diabetics' diet book: a new high-fibre eating programme.* Martin Dunitz, London.

Mattson, F.H. and Grundy, S.M. (1985). Comparison of effects of dietary saturated, monounsaturated, and polyunsaturated fatty acids on plasma lipids and lipoproteins in man. *J. Lipid Res.*, **19**, 194–202.

National Advisory Committee on Nutrition Education. (1983). *Proposals for nutritional guidelines for health education in Britain.* Health Education Council, London.

Report of the Committee on Medical Aspects of Food Policy. (1984). *Diet and cardiovascular disease.* DHSS report, HMSO, London.

Royal College of Physicians of London. (1980). *Report on medical aspects of dietary fibre.* Pitman Medical, London.

Thorogood, M., Carter, R., Benfield, L., McPherson, K., and Mann, J.I. (1987). Plasma lipids and lipoprotein cholesterol concentrations in people with different diets in Britain. *Brit. Med. J.*, **295**, 351–3.

Ulbricht, T. and Southgate, D.A.T. (1991) Coronary Heart Disease. Seven dietary factors. *Lancet*, **338**, 985–92.

Clinical trials—intervention

Ball, M. (1993). Dietary intervention trials—effect on cardiovascular morbidity and mortality. *Current Opinion in Lipidology*, **4**, 7–12.

Blankenhorn, D., *et al.* (1987). Beneficial effects of combined colestipol–niacin therapy on coronary atherosclerosis and coronary venous bypass of grafts. *JAMA*, **257**, 3233–40.

Brensike, J.F., Levy, R.I., Kelsey, S.F., *et al.* (1984). Effects of therapy with cholestyramine on progression of coronary atherosclerosis; results of the NHLBI type II coronary intervention study. *Circulation*, **69**, 313–24.

Brown, G. *et al.* (1990). Regression of coronary artery disease as a result of intensive lipid lowering therapy in men with high level of apolipoprotein B. *New Engl. J. Med.*, **323**, 1289–98.

Dayton, S., Pearce, M.L., Hashimoto, S., Dixon, W.J., and Tomiyasu, U. (1969). A controlled clinical trial of a diet high in unsaturated fat in preventing complications of atherosclerosis. *Circulation*, **40** (suppl. II), 58–60.

Duffield, R.G.M., Miller, N.E., Brunt, J.N.H., Lewis, B., Jamieson, C.W. and Colchester, A.C.F. (1983). Treatment of hyperlipidaemia retards progression of symptomatic femoral atherosclerosis. *Lancet*, **2**, 639–42.

Helsinki Heart Study. (1987). Primary prevention trial with gemfibrozil in middle-aged men with dyslipidemia. *New Engl. J. Med.* **317**, 1237–45.

Lipid Research Clinics Program (1984). Lipid Research Clinics Coronary Primary Prevention Trials Results. (1984). *JAMA*, **251**, 351–75.

Multiple Risk Factor Intervention Trial Research Group. (1982). Multiple Risk Factor Intervention Trial: Risk factor changes and mortality results. *JAMA*, **248**, 1465–77.

Nikkila, E.A., Viikiukoski, P., Valle, M., and Frick, M.H. (1984). Prevention of progression of coronary atherosclerosis by treatment of hyperlipidaemia: a seven-year prospective angiographic study. *Br. Med. J.*, **289**, 220–3.

Ornish, D., *et al.* (1990). Can lifestyle changes reverse coronary heart disease? *Lancet*, **336**, 129–33.

Peto, R., Yusuf, S., and Collins, R. (1987). Cholesterol-lowering trial results in their epidemiological context. *Circulation*, **75** (suppl. 2), 451.

Watts, G. *et al.* (1991). Effects on coronary artery disease of lipid lowering diet or diet plus cholestyramine in the St Thomas' Atherosclerosis Regression Study. *Lancet*, **339**, 563–9.

WHO (1980). Co-operative trial on primary prevention of ischaemic heart disease using clofibrate to lower serum cholesterol—mortality follow-up. *Lancet*, **ii**, 379–85.

WHO European Collaborative Group (1986). European collaborative trial of multifactorial prevention of coronary heart disease. *Lancet*, **1**, 869–72.

Articles

Angelin, B. and Rudling, M. (1992). Review—molecular aspects of human lipid metabolism. *Europ. J. Clin. Nutr.,* **42**, 153–60.

Anggard, E. (1986). Prevention of cardiovascular disease in general practice: a proposed model. *Brit. Med. J.*, **293**, 177–80.

Brown, M.S. and Goldstein, J.L. (1984). How LDL receptors influence choles-terol and atherosclerosis. *Sci. Am.*, **250**, 58–66.

Hoeg, J.M. Gregg, R.E., and Brewer, H.B. (1986). An approach to the manage-ment of hyperlipoproteinemia. *JAMA*, **255**, 512–22.

Jacobs, H. and Loeffer, F. (1992). Postmenopausal hormone replacement therapy. *Br. Med. J.*, **305**, 1403–8.

Lewis, B. (1983). The lipoproteins: predictors, protectors, and pathogens. *Brit. Med. J.*, **287**, 1161–3.

Lewis, B., Mann, J.I., and Mancini, M. (1986). Reducing the risks of coronary heart disease in individuals and in the population. *Lancet*, **1**, 956–9.

O'Conner, P., Feely, J. and Shepherd, J. (1990). Lipid lowering drugs. *Br. Med. J.*, **300**, 667–72.

Parthasarathy, S., Steinberg, D., and Witztum, J. (1992). The role of oxidised low-density lipoproteins in the pathogenesis of atherosclerosis. *Ann. Rev. Med.*, **43**, 219–25.

Royal College of Physicians of London (1983). Obesity. *J. Roy. Coll. Phys. Lond.*, **17**, 5–65.

Study Group, European Atherosclerosis Society (1987). Strategies for the pre-vention of coronary heart disease: A policy statement of the European Atherosclerosis Society. *Eur. Heart J.*, **8**, 77–88.

The British Cardiac Society Working Group on Coronary Prevention (1987). Conclusions and recommendations. *Brit. Heart. J.*, **57**, 188–9.

The management of hyperlipidaemia (1992). A consensus statement. *Med. J. Austr.*, **156**, 52–8.

United States Department of Health and Human Services (1983). *The health consequences of smoking: cardiovascular diseases. A report of the Surgeon General.* US Department of Health and Human Services, Public Health Service. DHHS (PHS) 84–50204.

Index

SOCIAL POLICY RESEARCH UNIT

Families Caring for People Diagnosed as Mentally Ill:
THE LITERATURE RE-EXAMINED

Christina Perring, Julia Twigg and Karl Atkin

London: HMSO

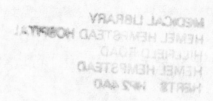
This Discussion Paper is based on work funded by Department of Health but
the opinions expressed are those of the researchers alone.

SPRU Editorial Group
Sally Baldwin
Lorna Foster
Gillian Parker
Roy Sainsbury
Patricia Thornton

Editor for this paper: Patricia Thornton

Acknowledgements

This review was prepared as part of the background to a larger research project concerned with evaluating support for informal carers. This, and its companion review, *Carers and Services: A Review of Research*, by J. Twigg, K. Atkin and C. Perring form the first publications of the research.

The project has been undertaken at the Social Policy Research Unit, University of York, and has been funded by the Department of Health. It forms part of a programme of work on informal care undertaken at the unit. Other publications in this field will appear as part of this HMSO/SPRU series. We would like to thank our many colleagues at SPRU for their helpful comments and suggestions. Particular thanks should go to Teresa Hagan, Gillian Parker and Patricia Thornton.

Contents

CHAPTER ONE

The scope of the review

The policy objectives of community care imply a major increase in responsibility for families with a member who has been diagnosed as mentally ill. Most recently, this has been underlined in the Government White Paper *Caring for People* (1989), with its continuing commitment to developing community-based services and the eventual closure of long-stay hospitals.

But what is it like to live with someone who is diagnosed as mentally ill? There are two obvious yet distinct bodies of research that address this issue. One is work in the field of informal care. The other, which is the principal focus of this paper, is found in the psychiatric and psychological literature. For various reasons, neither body of work adequately answers the question. Carers of people diagnosed as having a mental illness have been neglected in the main carer literature, which tends to concentrate on carers of people who require some physical tending. By contrast, literature in the psychiatric and psychological fields, which has developed quite separately, has tended to marginalise the position of carers, or 'relatives', in favour of concentrating on the well-being of the identified patient. Only rarely has this latter work looked at relatives in their own right.

This non-recognition of informal carers inspired this review. As part of a wider study seeking to evaluate support to informal carers, it was necessary to understand what it means to be a carer of someone diagnosed as mentally ill. For the most part, current attitudes to, and service intervention for, carers are moulded by notions of what a carer is that have been derived from the existing informal care literature. Caring for someone who experiences mental distress, however, is rather different from caring for someone who needs physical care. There is less emphasis on performing tasks, and caring is likely to vary with fluctuations in the course of the mental illness. The nature of the relationship and of responsibility is also subtly different. The dominant concept of informal care therefore has to be re-examined.

The ultimate aims of this paper are to reach an understanding of what life is like for carers of people diagnosed as mentally ill and to begin to relate this to what is already known about informal care.

Limitations of the literature

This review covers the research reported in the psychiatric and psychological literature that has investigated the impact of mental illness on families. This is a small body of work when compared with that on informal care or on community mental health in general. It appears to be the only body of work that addresses, albeit indirectly, the informal care of people diagnosed as mentally ill.

The scope of this literature is limited in a number of ways. Before discussing these and their consequences for our understanding of the situation of carers, we should perhaps indicate some of the limitations imposed on this review by ourselves. We have not, for example, included any discussion of the situation where the cared-for person is a child, or where the problem is one of substance abuse. Neither does the review include research about black carers. Race and mental health is an area now recognised to be of great importance, though it is also a controversial field and one neglected in the U.K. until relatively recently. There is as yet comparatively little published work, and the few studies reviewed here that do address race are from within an older, ethnocentric tradition that is dominated by white perceptions of health and family life. We felt that these situations raised specific issues that were inappropriate for this review. The review also excludes the carers of elderly mentally infirm people. Research in this field had been more successfully integrated with other work relating to elderly people and their carers; and for this reason the subject has been dealt with in the companion publication to this: *Carers and Services: A Review of Research* by Twigg, Atkin and Perring (1990).

The research perspective that underlies this review is one that attempts to place the carer, rather than the identified patient, at the centre of inquiry. It is important, therefore, to stress how little of the research reported here has taken that approach and investigated the situation of the carer per se. As a result, the writing of the review has itself been a creative process. It was necessary to re-orientate the literature and this has revealed a number of barriers to understanding. These arise from the character of the literature and inhibit its integration with the main carer work.

Barriers to understanding

There has inevitably been a strong medical influence in the fields of psychiatry and psychology. This can be seen, for instance, in the choice of topics for research, the methods chosen to investigate these topics and the language used to describe the findings. This medical focus has had implications for definitions and theories of mental illness and for the degree to which a single aspect of the patient has been treated as the object of inquiry (Armstrong, 1983; Atkin, 1989; Pearson, 1983). This has often been accompanied by a neglect of the more general non-medical, societal and familial aspects of mental illness such as those that have been examined in feminist or race analyses (see Chesler, 1972; Ineichen, 1989; Pearson, 1983). Only those aspects of the situation assumed to be directly related to a medical outcome have been seen as relevant.

The medical influence has also led to a particular emphasis on schizophrenia. This has been described as the prototypical example of 'mental illness' (Mechanic, 1986) and has traditionally been the preserve of the medical profession. Most of the studies reported here focus on families of patients diagnosed as schizophrenic; some do not differentiate between diagnoses and only a few have focused on families of depressed people. As a result, our understanding of the situation is heavily biased towards the problems of schizophrenia. This imbalance of focus makes it hard to examine the differential impact on families of different psychiatric states. It is difficult, for example, to determine whether, and if so how, the situation of caring for someone who is clinically depressed differs from that of caring for someone who is diagnosed as schizophrenic.

The methodological approaches adopted in the fields of psychiatry and psychology have been largely influenced by those of the natural sciences. As a result, there has been an emphasis in this work on quantitative methodology, and it has been seen as appropriate to examine the situation in terms of variables and statistical rela-tionships. Different aspects of family life are separated into variables, which are then measured or assessed. Researchers have, however, tended to use idiosyncratic measures and it is often difficult to draw direct comparisons across the research, since each study tends to conceptualise the situation somewhat differently. This is particularly so where 'global' measures of impact are generated by combining variables in ways that are particular to the research project. Little attention has been paid to the meaning of the situation for individual carers and to their interpretation of it. The situation is most frequently conceptualised within the rather limited framework of 'burden' and the complexity of the interactions and feelings have not been very intensively explored.

The language used to describe the findings both reflects and frames the orientations adopted. The language of informal care refers to disability, cared-for person, dependant, carer. The world of mental health refers to illness, patient, relative or supporter. The different assumptions that underlie this choice of language, as well as the language itself, have hampered the process of interpretation.

In addition to the barriers that arise in relating findings across different disciplines, there are perspectives within disciplines that pose barriers to understanding. Emphasis on the well-being of families in its own right is only a comparatively recent interest in the field. More usually, interest in the well-being of families has been only for its significance as a means to the greater end of helping the patient.

This general lack of attention to family well-being was highlighted as early as 1968 (Grad and Sainsbury, 1968). Some more recent reviews, such as that by Keisler (1982), include only a brief reference to families; the updated version (1984) of Talbott's influential book devotes only one of its 22 chapters to the families of chronic mental patients. This is despite the fact that 60 per cent of first-episode schizophrenic patients live with their families (MacCarthy, Kuipers, Hurry, Harper and LeSage, 1989a). Although Fadden, Bebbington and Kuipers (1987a) described this as a large body of literature, it remains unsatisfactory with regard to its coverage of, and relevance to, carers.

That the literature is unsatisfactory comes, in part, from the fact that there are distinct themes in the literature on families and mental health. Gubman and Tessler (1987) have described three of these, all of which show bias in their interest towards favourable outcome for the patient. These themes are the role of the family in both the origins of mental distress and rehabilitation, and what has become known as 'family burden'. Much of the research on the first two themes has been influenced by a perception of the family as having a potentially pathogenic influence on mental illness (e.g. Laing and Esterson, 1964/1982; Vaughn and Leff, 1976). Although the influence of this perspective has waned, there is a risk that aspects of it may inappropriately have been carried over into the third theme, that of family burden.

More recently, a change in orientation has taken place. This has occurred against the policy background of increased care in the community, as well as an increased interest in the carer generally. It is now more common to view the family as a source of support and care (Kreisman and Joy, 1974; Vaughn and Leff, 1981) and some attention has been paid to ways of enhancing this family role (Crotty and Kulys, 1986; Hawks, 1975). Some recent work has focused on families as coping with and adapting to the impact of mental illness (Hatfield and Lefley, 1987; Orford, 1987), though even this work is more concerned with developing a 'non-blaming stance' towards families, rather than with placing them at the centre of inquiry. Little work that maintains this latter focus has been reported.

It is difficult to abstract from the body of work under review any sense of what life is like for a carer of someone identified as having mental illness. This is seen, for instance, in major reviews of the literature where the principal focus has been on the effect of relatives on patients' well-being, rather than on the effect of the situation on families or carers themselves (Braun, Kochansky, Shapiro, Greenberg, Goudeman, Johnson and Shore, 1981; Fadden et al., 1987a; Kreisman and Joy, 1974). Most studies recognise that caring takes place within the context of family relationships but have tended to examine the effect of caring only in terms of disruption to different aspects of family life, known as 'family burden'. This provides a rather restricted view of the situation, and one that is in contrast to that presented in the main carer literature where more complex notions of the caring role have been developed.

Lastly, the mental health literature emphasises the impact on the family as a whole, rather than on individual carers. The carer literature suggests, however, that the caring responsibility is rarely shared and that a single individual tends to carry most of that responsibility (Parker, 1990). In the mental health literature, this sharper focus is blurred.

Conclusion

There are a number of characteristics of this literature that pose barriers to our understanding of this situation. These also act as obstacles to integrating this understanding with the literature on informal care. Emphasis has been on families, rather than on individuals, involved in a situation which is seen as one of 'burden' rather than as one of informal care. The medical interest that has influenced this work has tended to focus on the well-being of the patient, and on people diagnosed as schizophrenic. Methods of inquiry have neglected the meaning of the situation to those concerned. These differences of emphasis are rooted mainly in the different assumptions and perspectives that underlie the two distinct bodies of work. By examining these and reorientating the findings, we can begin to answer the question posed at the beginning of this chapter: 'What is it like to live with someone who is diagnosed as mentally ill?'.

The core of this review is devoted to three main areas of inquiry. Chapter Two examines the impact on the family; this includes a discussion of the research on what has become known as 'family burden'. Chapter Three considers why the impact of caring may be more difficult for some people than for others. A review of families and service provision follows in Chapter Four.

Impact on family life

In the psychiatric and psychological literature, the tasks performed by the family, the particular features of mental illness and the impact of both of these on family life have all become known as 'family burden'. Research evidence from different disciplines shows that the task of caring is likely to be burdensome. Conceptualisations of the situation that exclude more complex patterns of response are likely to provide only a partial representation of the situation. There have been only minor moves away from such narrow conceptualisations of the caring situation in the psychiatric and psychological literature. Creer, Sturt and Wykes (1982), for instance, have proposed that the term 'burden' be replaced by the more neutral term 'support'. In doing so, they implicitly recognise that the role of caring encompasses a slightly wider range of experience that may include the more positive aspects of a relationship. The dominant model, as in the rest of the carer literature, is that of 'family burden'. In this paper, we have sought to avoid some of the more negative and restrictive connotations of this by using the term 'impact'.

It is from this area of research that links can most readily be made to the main literature on carers, where the effect of caring for elderly people or those with disabilities, for instance, has been well documented (Parker 1990).

The caring tasks

Before turning to the different aspects of family life that are affected by caring, we describe the caring tasks themselves. These can be grouped into three main categories: practical tasks, coping with difficult behaviour and new responsibilities.

Practical tasks

Very few studies have provided good data on what carers of people diagnosed as mentally ill do. They have tended to emphasise the impact of caring on family life, rather than the detail of the caring task. This is in contrast to what is known about those caring for disabled people. One study that has detailed the range of tasks performed by carers was that of Creer et al. (1982). They divided their 18 items of what relatives do for dependants into the practical tasks that people are normally expected to do for themselves; the types of behaviour that might need supervision from the carer; and whether the dependent person can be left alone. As might be expected, relatively few of their 52 patients with mixed psychiatric diagnoses required help with washing and dressing. However, over half had some difficulty with household chores or needed help with financial arrangements. Medication was also an area where supervision was needed. In all, three quarters of relatives reported that at least some 'caring attention' was necessary with regard to socially difficult aspects of the patients' behaviour, which included serious attention-seeking behaviour, threats or violence, night disturbance, and carers being unable to leave the house unattended for longer than a few hours at a time.

Tasks were principally those of assuming responsibility for their dependant in various ways, rather than of giving practical help. In this respect, caring for someone diagnosed as mentally ill tends to be rather different from caring for someone with a physical disability where personal care or other practical help is usually an essential part of the care being provided. In some ways, it may be more like the care afforded to people with learning difficulties, who cannot assume full responsibility for their lives. However, with regard to mental illness, the need both to provide practical help and to assume responsibility fluctuates with the course of the illness. Another important difference is in the nature of the relationship between dependant and carer. The onset of mental illness typically occurs once the dependant has reached adolescence or adulthood, unlike the situation for a dependant with learning difficulties whose need for care is likely to have existed since birth.

Coping with difficult behaviour
Coping with the behaviour associated with mental illness is difficult for carers, just as it is for members of society as a whole. In many cases, it is this aspect of the situation that poses most problems for carers. Even so, few studies have described these behaviours in terms of what they mean to carers. What frequently happens is that a form of shorthand is used to identify clusters of behaviour. This refers to clinical terms like 'withdrawal' or 'florid symptoms', without explaining what the implications of these might be for carers.

Creer (1975) is unusual in providing a description of the sorts of behaviour with which carers have to contend, although she also tends to resort to this clinical shorthand. She reports how carers faced with a relapse of their relative diagnosed as schizophrenic see an increase of the behaviour typically associated with the syndrome. This might mean an increase both in social withdrawal and in behaviour that is described as 'more florid'. Social withdrawal is exemplified by people who shut themselves in their own rooms for hours or even days and, having lost the confidence to seek social life outside the home, became increasingly demanding of their family. This can act as a severe constraint on the carer's own life, especially when he or she feels unable to leave his or her relative. Neglect of appearance and cleanliness is common. Uncontrollable restlessness is one of the most disturbing examples of the more florid types of behaviour. Here, carers face behavioural difficulties similar to those shown by people with Alzheimer's Disease. These can include excessive activity such as pacing the room or, for younger adults, playing loud music at night. Such activity causes friction both in the family and with neighbours. The strong beliefs that dependent relatives may hold at such periods also cause difficulties for the carer. Creer gives examples of one patient who believed that 'he was being controlled by a hypnotist, and another that he and his family were being slowly poisoned' (p.3).

People who are depressed, whether or not this is associated with schizophrenia, show a range of behaviour that includes threatened, attempted or actual suicide, withdrawn behaviour with no incli-nation to speak, and frustrating hypochondriacal preoccupations (Grad and Sainsbury 1963). Social withdrawal and 'quiet misery' are common. Relatives have frequently reported these 'negative' symp-toms as being more difficult to cope with than the more florid symptoms of schizophrenia (Creer and Wing, 1974; Vaughn, 1977, cited in Fadden et al, 1987a). There may be a tendency to ascribe attitudes like this to the identified patient's character, and see him or her as 'selfish' or 'lazy' (Vaughn, 1977 cited in Fadden et al, 1987a). This appears to make coping with a depressed relative especially difficult, as he or she, rather than depressive illness, is blamed:

> whereas relatives are apprehensive of florid symptoms, it is the suppressive effects of mental illness on behaviour that cause the most problems, and this is partly due to the difficulty which relatives have in attributing such effects to mental illness.
> (Fadden et al., 1987a, p.288)

These behaviours also left carers uncertain about how to respond. Creer reported that carers did not know whether to encourage sociability or to allow relatives to withdraw further. They did not want to be unsympathetic towards their relatives, but felt frustrated and baffled by bizarre behaviour. Embarrassment in public over their relatives' behaviour was common among carers. It appeared that carers found it easier to cope with stable rather than fluctuating, and with florid rather than withdrawn behaviour.

New responsibilities

The resurgence of symptoms often means that the relative is unable to cope with many practical details of everyday life, from personal care to household and financial responsibilities and personal relationships. The carer is at this point likely to have to assume a new role with regard to responsibilities. This may involve supervision of the dependant and the conduct of household roles. This new role is likely to be affected by the kin relationship between carer and dependant. A spouse confronted by the need to make financial decisions or to become the principal breadwinner is in a different position from the parent of an adult child who may be reverting to an earlier pattern of relationship. The change may be experienced differently by men and women, and by younger and older carers.

One study that recognised this shift with regard to spouse carers was that of Fadden, Bebbington and Kuipers (1987b). This small scale, though intensive, study examined the impact of caring for 24 spouses of depressed patients. The researchers related the impact of caring to what people expect from the reciprocal relationships that are seen as integral to family life. This aspect of family life may differ according to the particular kin relationship involved, although until recently the literature on informal care had tended to neglect the role of these differences (but see Parker, 1989, for a comprehensive study of spouse carers, and Finch, 1989, for an examination of family obligations).

Fadden et al.'s spouse carers had to take over many household responsibilities at a time when they were also experiencing the much felt loss of a confiding relationship. What Fadden and her colleagues were examining, however, was not so much the assumption of responsibility itself, but its presumed connection to role change within the family. Role changes and role conflict have been reported in other carer studies where high levels of role strain have been found, and relatives reported a need to increase their supervision of relatives because of difficult behaviour (Thompson and Doll, 1982).

These issues have also been examined in other literature concerned with carers. For instance, the loss of functioning that accompanies diseases such as Alzheimer's Disease, Huntington's Chorea (Korer and Fitzsimmons, 1985) or head injury also result in role changes. Related to this is the acute sense of loss and bereavement for the person whose changed behaviour is so extensive that the carer feels as though they are living with a completely different person. 'As one mother put it, "You just can't understand it. Here's someone you've known all these years and always got on well with, and suddenly he can't even stand being in the same room with you"' (Creer, 1975, p.4). Carers have to come to terms both with a shift in responsibility and with the loss of the person they knew.

It seems likely that when someone assumes the role of carer there will be permanent shifts in family roles and considerable unanticipated responsibility falling consistently to one carer. Studies appear to have neglected precise descriptions of such shifts in responsibility. This is likely to be related to, among other things, assumptions about relationships and to the neglect of possible differences between them.

Disruption to family life

Research on the impact on family life has looked at different areas such as marital and parental relationships, domestic routine, social life, leisure activity, employment, financial circumstances, and various aspects of health. Many studies have combined these aspects in different ways to produce a single 'global' measure of the situation. Platt (1985, Table 1) details criteria for evaluating burden scales. This is comprehensive and methodologically clear and provides a good illustration of the approach adopted in this body of research.

He identifies ten areas of family life that may be affected by caregiving and distinguishes these from the eleventh area of burden, impact directly attributable to the patient's behaviour. Sexual functioning is the only additional area that can be added from other studies reported here (Fadden et al., 1987a; Namyslowska, 1986). Platt's four dimensions of burden explicitly separate elements of the situation often confounded or overlooked in other studies, while his list of people to whom burden relates recognises the differential impact of experience for people within the household and outside it.

Most studies have reported considerable overall levels of disruption to family life where someone diagnosed as being mentally ill is being cared for. Thompson and Doll (1982) found that nearly three quarters of their 125 family caregivers were adversely affected by disruption to family life in at least one of five different areas. Johnstone, Owens, Gold, Crow and MacMillan (1984) used what they described as an arbitrary list of seven items to measure the overall impact on family life. Thirteen of their 42 informants reported no difficulties, while 18 'gave positive answers to at least three items' (p.587), indicating

Table 1   *Typology of burden* (drawn from Platt, 1985)

Eleven areas of burden
Effect on
   work/employment
   social life, leisure
   physical health
   emotional/mental health
   finances/income
   family routine
   family/household interaction
   schooling/education
   children
   (interaction with) others outside the household/family
Patient's behaviour as a burden

Four dimensions of burden
Objective burden, which may be rated
   if present, regardless of 'cause'
   if present, and only if attributable to patient
Subjective burden
   arising directly out of patient's behaviour
   arising as a consequence of (increased) objective burden

Five persons to whom burden relates
Informant
Specific others in household
Informant's household as a totality
Specific others outside the household
Non-specific others outside the informant's household (e.g.
   community)

major difficulties. In a study with spouses of depressed patients, Fadden et al. (1987b) also found that relatives bear burdens that are far-reaching in many areas of their lives. They cite the high incidence of marital breakdown among families with a schizophrenic member as further evidence for this claim.

None of these studies included a comparison or control group. It is therefore difficult to be certain that the reported difficulties are associated with mental illness in the family and are not a feature of 'normal' family life. One study that did use a control group was that conducted in Poland by Namyslowska (1986). She found few differences in family functioning between research (those containing a schizophrenic member) and control families. One difference, however, was that research families spent their free time in more home-based pursuits; just over one third of research families saw this as due to the schizophrenic illness of the spouse. Another major difference was that fewer children from such homes participated in extra school activities. Other areas of family life, such as the economic, caretaking and educational, did not differ significantly between research and control families. The large number of families (1,832) used to establish normal levels of functioning in her study suggests it is unlikely that undetected psychiatric disturbance has contributed to the lack of difference between the two sets of families.

McCreadie, Wiles, Moore, Grant et al. (1987) compared scores for families with a member experiencing a first episode of schizophrenia (research families) with norms derived from a community sample. They found that research families scored significantly worse on global adjustment and social and leisure function, but better on parental functioning. These measures were scored on a 54-item questionnaire that provides an overall rating and a rating in each of seven role areas (the Social Adjustment Scale Self-Report, Weissman and Bothwell, 1976, cited in McCreadie et al., 1987).

Bromet, Ed and May (1984) found that, for families with a depressed adult, family functioning was affected only while the depressed adult was experiencing current symptoms. At that time, higher levels of marital conflict were reported in research than in control families, although this conflict did not extend to family relationships as a whole.

These studies show that, on an overall assessment of disruption to family life, many families experience considerable difficulty when they live with someone identified as mentally ill. Taken together, they are important in establishing the types of disturbance that may occur. Nevertheless, there has been a tradition in research on mental health, from Freud to the present day, of investigating only those families where disturbance is apparent. There is a need to set findings from this tradition in a context of evidence from 'normal' families, where the experience of possibly severe disturbance has also been reported.

There are aspects of the situation that remain unexamined in these studies. First, there is no clear description of what life is like for individual carers. This literature sets out to describe what the impact is like for the family as a whole, and rarely pays attention to the impact on individual family members. In particular, this means that the impact for the primary carer has not generally been addressed. Second, little attention is paid to the fact that the course of mental illness fluctuates, and periods of intensive caring may be broken by several months or years where the identified patient leads a symptom-free life. Fadden and her colleagues (1987b) hinted at this aspect of psychiatric distress when they commented that many of their interviews with the spouses of patients with manic depression were conducted when the patient was asymptomatic. This means that many reported findings cannot be taken to be representative of what life is like during periods of crisis. This is a major methodological difficulty in the literature.

Social and personal life

The most common finding among studies of families with a psychiatrically ill member was that social life was restricted or disrupted (Fadden et al. 1987b; Johnstone et al., 1984). This complements the findings of McCreadie et al. and Namyslowska who found a difference between control and research families with regard to leisure activities. Fadden et al.'s study is important because it concerned depressed people. She reported that particular distress for family members was associated with restricted social activity. This parallels the experience of restrictedness in the main carer literature. Further evidence for disruption to social life is found in studies that report problems with neighbours and role strain (Thompson and Doll, 1982), disruption of family relationship (Johnstone et al., 1984) and global adjustment (McCreadie et al. 1987). In addition, it is in recreational and cultural activities outside the home that research and control families show the most significant difference in functioning (Namyslowska, 1986).

One of the few studies that gives a sense of what happens to the social life of individual carers is by Fadden et al. (1987b). Spouses objected to the 'smothering' nature of the relationship that followed from a curtailment of social and recreational activity and isolation from friends. In addition, some studies have included brief descriptions that provide an impression of this and other aspects of the situation for individual carers (Creer, 1975). Again, there are parallels to be drawn with studies that have looked at the spouse carers of disabled adults where the loss of stimulating external social contact is widespread (Parker, 1989).

Most studies show that major sources of social support are severely restricted for carers, and loss of social life is frequently reported as one of the most distressing aspects of the situation. This clearly fits with Brown and Harris' (1978) view of the importance of close confiding relationships in protecting against depression. For many carers, close relationships are denied. In addition to the impact on their social life, they may be caring for a close relative who might normally be expected to be a source of emotional support. Spouse carers seem particularly likely to lose their major confiding relationship given that the nature of many forms of mental illness means that the identified patient is no longer able to offer such support to the carer.

Employment and financial circumstances

The impact of caring on employment is not uniform. Fadden and her colleagues (1987b) reported that few carers had had to make changes to their work routine, though work was reported as a strain by half of their interviewees and two women had taken up full time employment for financial reasons. Reduced performance at work was reported by 80 per cent of relatives interviewed by Gibbons, Horn, Powell and Gibbons (1984), while nearly half of the families in Johnstone et al.'s (1984) study had been affected either by giving up works or by taking time off to care. While it is clear from these studies that the proportions of people having to make changes to their employment pattern as a result of mental illness in the family is small, there are other effects, such as increased strain, which interviewees do relate to their employment role.

The nature of the tasks that characterise caring for someone with mental illness – responsibility as against physical tending, and fluctuating as against constant care – may lead to the supposition that carers in this situation will find it more feasible to combine caring and employment. The mainstream literature on informal care, however, has pointed to a complex relationship between gender, unpaid caregiving and paid employment. This relationship also encompasses other aspects of the situation such as household composition and marital status (Glendinning, 1989). We can draw no firm conclusions about the employment of this group of carers until adequate research has been conducted, but we can assume that any relationship between caring and employment is likely to be equally as complex as that reported in the carer literature.

The situation with regard to financial circumstances is clearer. The majority of studies that have investigated the financial situation have found difficulties which carers related directly to the presence of mental illness in the family. Thompson and Doll (1982) and Gibbons et al. (1984) both found very similar proportions of households were adversely affected (38 and 39 per cent respectively). Fadden et al. (1987b) found that for a large percentage of households, financial problems were reported as much worse since the spouse had become ill. Financial difficulties were often due to loss of income when the male breadwinner was unable to continue in paid employment (Johnstone et al., 1984). Again, Glendinning's work has shown complex patterns of financial consequences, which vary with, among other things, household composition.

Emotional impact

In addition to the tasks to be performed and their effect on family routine, researchers have also investigated how families respond emotionally to different aspects of the situation. Both this, and those aspects of the situation that are less amenable to quantitative measurement, have usually been referred to as 'subjective burden' in the literature. Most studies have sought to identify those aspects of the situation that are sources of the more negative emotional responses. Within a quantitative framework, this has been predominantly through correlational studies. While this approach may show that two aspects of a situation are associated, it does not necessarily establish either causality or the direction of any causal relationship that is established. It is therefore limited in its explanatory power. We describe the emotions that have been identified in different studies, before examining the correlates of these emotions.

A wide range of emotional responses to mental illness occurring in a family member has been identified in the literature. Kreisman and Joy (1974) showed that these have mostly been negative or upsetting, but occasionally they have included positive responses. Feelings of marginalisation, fear of the patient, anger and resentment and shame are common. On the other hand, more positive feelings of warmth and love for the dependant have also been reported (Gillis and Keet, 1965, cited in Kreisman and Joy; Namyslowska, 1986).

Thompson and Doll (1982) investigated some of the feelings that relatives might be expected to have. They used four main indicators – feelings of being overloaded, of being trapped, of resentment and of exclusion (or the need to withdraw from the patient). The most common feeling was of being overloaded. This they defined as being where there was 'a significant interference to the family and a noticeable emotional drain' (p.382). Nearly one half of their relatives reported feeling embarrassed and, in a separate measure, feeling trapped. Resentment and bitterness were expressed by 40 per cent of their sample; for 13 per cent of the sample, this bitterness was intense. Some need to withdraw from the patient was expressed by nearly one third of relatives, though very few (7 per cent) wished for greater social distance from the identified patient.

Creer, Sturt and Wykes (1982) used measures of satisfaction, resignation and dissatisfaction to assess the impact of supporting mentally ill relatives at home. The researchers first identified through detailed questioning specific responsibilities and tasks performed during the month prior to interview. They then assessed the emotional response to each task and made an overall rating. Nearly two thirds of relatives were content with their caring and household responsibilities, even when these were extensive. However, relatives frequently expressed a need for emotional support in coping with their own feelings and their reactions to the patient's behaviour and illness. Specific emotions reported were guilt, associated with the relatives blaming themselves for the patient's condition, and emotional exhaustion. 'With few exceptions, the research team concluded that relatives' complaints were not only justified but understated' (p.38).

This study recognises a slightly wider range of emotional response (from satisfaction to dissatisfaction) than many other studies. It thus includes the more positive responses to caring. By using the category 'resigned', these researchers have also recognised that relatives may have come to terms with a difficult situation. Conceptualisations of the caring role generally neglect or overlook the fact that the situation is too stressful to be seen as 'satisfactory', but that carers may nevertheless have come to accept the role as the best or only option available to them.

Many studies have shown a variety of unpleasant emotional experiences for relatives. Only a few have moved towards concept-ualising caring as encompassing more pleasant emotional experi-ences. These experiences may be more prevalent than the literature suggests. However, it seems more likely that the dominant emotional responses are unpleasant.

In addition to providing details of the range of emotional experience, researchers have sought to identify specific aspects of the situation that are associated with these emotions. Kreisman and Joy (1974) concluded that shame and fear are as likely to be associated with unrestrained behaviour as with the formal labelling of the patient. Shame and perception of stigma have behavioural consequences too, such as a need for secrecy or concealment and withdrawal from friends. Practical considerations, such as the duration of the illness or number of hospital admissions, inevitably affect efforts to conceal what is felt to be a shameful family situation. Other clinical aspects of the situation that affect the family are considered in Chapter Three.

For a majority of relatives there is an association between emotional distress and the more measurable aspects of the situation. Gibbons et al. (1984) interviewed 143 schizophrenic patients and 166 people who supported them. In 90 per cent of households, these relatives or friends experienced distress caused by friction due to a variety of reasons. Financial hardship, reduced performance at work, physical ill health and disruption outside the household 'were distressing to 80 per cent of those affected' (p.75). Namyslowska (1986) found that 64 per cent of relatives believed schizophrenic illness in the family had affected their emotional life in some way. While some spouses reported that the illness had 'cemented their love', most people reported negative emotional responses in respect of changes in economic, educational and emotional functioning. The strongest negative emotional responses concerned change in the areas of recreational and sexual functioning and in feelings of security.

Studies have also sought links between distressing emotions and aspects of the situation that are less amenable to measurement. Creer (1975) found that emotional distress among relatives was related to fears for the future, frustration with the current unchanging situation, loss of the schizophrenic relative's 'former self' and a sense of failure as a parent. Some respondents reported a sense of guilt that could be exacerbated when professional workers attributed blame to the parenting. Creer concludes that, although such emotional responses are 'normal' reactions to a confusing situation, they can impair the ability of the carer to cope with the situation. Other studies, such as those by Creer, Sturt and Wykes (1982), Namyslowska (1986), and Seymour and Dawson (1986) confirm these findings that relatives identify the less easily measured aspects of the situation as being more closely associated with emotional distress than the more easily quantifiable features such as financial or educational disruption.

The dominant quantitative method of the literature under review often pays more attention to the more easily measured aspects of family life and less attention to issues of interpretation and meaning. However, the literature in general suggests that it is the more subtle and personal concerns (of losing a close relationship or anxieties for the individual's future) that are the aspects of the situation that cause greatest emotional distress to carers. Emphasis is not so much on tasks to perform as on difficulties to be managed or tolerated. Carers are thus placed in a position where they need to cope with long term difficulties. Despite this, the general literature on coping with stress has not been applied either to the family experience of mental illness specifically (Avison and Speechley, 1987) or to personal welfare at a more general level (Titterton, 1989). This is likely to be a fruitful area for future research, and is discussed more fully in Chapter Five.

Physical and psychiatric health

Another way of assessing families' response to the caring situation has been to use physical and psychiatric health as indicators. Again, studies have often used correlations to examine associations between health and different aspects of the caring situation.

One study that examined physical health was that of Creer (1975). She reported that less than 20 per cent of her sample of carers of schizophrenic relatives showed no impairment of physical health or well-being. One third showed a 'very severe' degree of impairment. Gibbons et al. (1984) found that nearly three quarters of relatives showed symptoms of physical or psychiatric ill health, as measured by the Social Behaviour Assessment Schedule (SBAS, Platt et al., 1980, cited in Gibbons et al.). This study, however, reports no further details about physical health.

The provisos raised by Parker (1990) are pertinent here when assessing the impact of caring on physical health. Problems of physical health increase with age, so that, 'as the General Household Survey shows around two thirds of people over the age of 45 report chronic health problems' (p. 53). Many people diagnosed as mentally ill are cared for by their parents, and it is likely that age is an important correlate with the carer's physical health. It is not always clear whether deterioration in health can be directly attributed to the caring role. Studies reported by Parker among elderly carers and mothers of handicapped children suggest that caring is not necessarily responsible, nor seen as responsible by carers, for a decline in health. Class, race and gender are other variables that affect health, though these have not been investigated rigorously in this body of literature. More detailed investigations are needed before firm conclusions can be made about links between physical health and caring for someone diagnosed as mentally ill. These will need to consider such aspects of the situation as age, socio-economic class, race and gender of the carer and also whether ill health can be properly attributed to the caring role.

It has been more common for researchers to investigate psychiatric distress than physical health among carers. As has been mentioned above, Gibbons et al. (1984) found that nearly three quarters of relatives showed symptoms of psychiatric or physical ill health, though their report does not differentiate between the two as measured by the SBAS. Relatives living with patients diagnosed for less than one year were more likely to show higher rates of psychiatric distress as measured by the General Health Questionnaire (GHQ). Nearly one half of these scored above the threshold that indicates a level of symptoms severe enough to suggest clinical disturbance. Overall, one third of relatives showed symptoms of this intensity. In addition, the Scottish First Episode Schizophrenia Study (McCreadie et al., 1987) found that relatives scored approximately three times higher than the community norm on the GHQ, showing a very high level of psychiatric distress. These studies, and other work such as that of Hirsch and Leff (1975), have shown that families with a mentally ill member experience levels of psychiatric distress that are more severe than those considered normal on the basis of community norms. Both of these studies also found that psychiatric distress among family members was associated with the patient's clinical status. A detailed analysis of the relevant aspects of clinical status is reported more fully in Chapter Three.

Other variables have also been shown to be associated with psychiatric distress in relatives. McCreadie et al. (1987) found that where symptoms were most severe, the relative was more likely to have poorer social adjustment, and poorer functioning both within the nuclear family and at work. Distress is generally greater where there is a shorter history of caring for someone with mental illness, as for someone with dementia (Gilhooly, 1984). Gibbons et al. (1984) have suggested that this reflects families' abilities to adapt to coping with the situation. There are other possible explanations. The early period of caring, before adjustment has taken place, has often been identified as particularly stressful. Relatives who have recently experienced the trauma of diagnosis may be showing the sort of distress known to follow life events (Brown and Harris, 1978). In addition, those families that do not cope do not remain intact. They are thus excluded from studies based on surviving families.

Studies such as these that use measures like the GHQ may underestimate symptom levels over prolonged periods of time. The measure assesses how respondents have been feeling during the previous two weeks compared with how they normally feel. If the caring situation has existed for several years, the baseline of what is normal may be different from situations where caring has been taking place only for weeks or months. This is a point emphasized by Parker (1990). She showed that as carers become used to the caring role, they may cease to regard the situation as unusually stressful and may overlook deterioration in health that has occurred over a long period of time. What is clear is that those families that do survive intact do so in part because they are able to accommodate to a distressing situation, but probably only at a cost of higher than normal levels of psychiatric distress.

Conclusion

Overall, despite conceptual difficulties and methodological diversity, there is among researchers some consensus both about the extent of impact and about the types of experience and behaviour that can be said to constitute and produce it. What is less clear is precisely whether and, if so, how this differs from the disturbance in 'normal' families. Platt's question of whether disturbance is attributable to the presence of a psychiatrically distressed person is highly relevant.

The question is not only whether other family members attribute disturbance to one individual, but also whether disturbance should be attributed to the presence of mental illness at all. 'Normal' family disturbance may risk being seen as pathological where a member has been labelled as psychiatrically ill and has become drawn into the service system. This may result in disturbance being mistakenly attributed to the mental illness of one individual. Studies that include control or comparison groups will help to clarify this issue. Finally, many gaps in basic knowledge remain about the impact of living with someone with psychiatric distress especially when it is remembered that most studies have focused on people with schizophrenia rather than other forms of mental illness.

CHAPTER THREE

What makes caring more difficult for some than for others?

There are some characteristics of the caring situation that mean that difficulties are greater for some carers than for others. Personal characteristics that have been reported include socio-demographic variables, such as kin relationship, age and gender of the carer; clinical characteristics of the identified patient; and social support of both the family and the identified patient. In this body of work, however, characteristics such as age, gender and kin relationship have often been confounded. There is a need for studies that tease out such characteristics properly.

Kin relationship

There is growing interest in the main carer literature in how caring is constructed differently in different situations. One of the ways in which we increasingly refine the concept of carer is with regard to kin relationship. Important differences have been identified between, for instance, spouse and parental relationships (Parker, 1989).

Most studies that have investigated kin relationship between carer and dependant report no association between any particular kin relationship and increased strain for the carer (Gibbons et al., 1984; McCreadie et al. 1987; Seymour and Dawson, 1986; Thompson and Doll, 1982). These studies have examined a number of variables and related these to measures of distress and health. However, what they show is that, not surprisingly, relatives report different sorts of concern according to the kin relationship. Parents are concerned about the future care of their offspring, while spouses are distressed by changes in the marital role. This can be compared to findings in the main carer literature.

The range of kin relationships has not been systematically explored. Many studies (particularly the earlier ones such as those of Yarrow and Clausen and their co-workers, 1955) focused on wives caring for husbands and cannot be said adequately to have separated out the differences between issues of gender and issues of kin relationship.

Many people who develop mental illness do not marry (Cheadle, Freeman and Korer, 1978) while some relationships, such as those between siblings, are less likely to develop into caring ones. In addition, studies sometimes confound problems specific to kin relationships with those of co-residence (Gubman and Tessler, 1987).

The studies that show there is no differential impact with kin relationship may reflect the fact that measures of overall impact have been used. There is a need to use methods that are sensitive enough to assess those strains that are specific to particular kin relationships, and it is likely that only a specifically designed study will provide appropriate research material. So far as we are aware, this type of study has not been conducted. Those of Fadden et al. (1987b) and Rogler and Hollingshead (1965) were conducted with spouses only, and were not designed specifically to investigate gender differences even within this relationship. In addition, Rogler and Hollingshead's study was conducted among Puerto Ricans, and the possibility of differences with regard to racial and cultural characteristics has not been disentangled from differences with regard to gender or kin relationship. It is not possible to say definitively, for instance, whether spouses are more adversely affected than parents. This is an area where considerably more research is needed.

Age

The issue of age is particularly relevant given the common pattern of responsibility of parents caring for mentally ill offspring. The position of single dependent adults living with ageing parents has been highlighted as a particular problem (Braun et al., 1981; Creer and Wing, 1974; Seymour and Dawson 1986; Stevens, 1972). Stevens has also shown how this situation may benefit both carer and dependant, for the elderly parents may gain from the company of their adult offspring. This may be particularly so for an elderly widow. She points out that this type of caring relationship may offer an important source of social cohesion when the more usual family pattern is for adult offspring to move away from the family of origin and have little day to day contact with an ageing relative. However, there are also difficulties inherent in this situation. A frequent cause for anxiety among ageing relatives is the continuation of suitable care once they themselves are unable to offer daily support; and this type of symbiotic relationship may inhibit the dependant from living more independently in the community.

On the other hand, those investigations that have included age among a range of socio-demographic variables have shown no relationship between age and the impact of caring. These include the studies of Gibbons et al. (1984) and Thompson and Doll (1982). It is possible that where issues concerned with age are specifically investigated, then particular difficulties are identified – fears for the future or a symbiotic relationship that may inhibit independent living. However, such difficulties when measured within a quantitative framework may appear to present no greater difficulties for ageing parents than difficulties concerning the well-being of school age children present to younger carers. The findings on age may more usefully contribute towards an understanding of those aspects of the caring situation that are most salient at a particular stage of family history, rather than demonstrating that the role of caring is more stressful for older than for younger carers. It is clear that the diverse situations of carers present diverse difficulties. It seems likely that contradictory findings reported in the literature reflect this diversity.

Gender

A similarly mixed pattern of results is seen when gender of the carer is considered. Studies by Gibbons et al. (1984), McCreadie et al. (1987) and Thompson and Doll (1982) have shown that gender of the carer is not associated with differences in the impact of caring. Some studies of spousal relationships have shown that greater family disruption is found where wives are the carers (Fadden et al., 1987b; Namyslowska, 1986). Others have shown that disruption is greater where husbands are the carers (Rogler and Hollingshead, 1965). Mandlebrote and Folkard (1961) reported that where women were caring, disruption was greater in the conjugal rather than the parental role (cited in Fadden et al., 1987b).

Crotty and Kulys (1986) found a marked difference between the perceptions of male and female relatives. Nearly two thirds of the 39 women they interviewed did not see caring for a man as a burden. In contrast, nearly two thirds of their 17 male carers did see the situation as burdensome. The authors interpret this as being consistent with the way women are socialised in the United States, where the study took place. In Poland, Namyslowska (1986) found that men and women adopted different coping strategies. Men were 'inclined to denial' while women were 'looking for information even at the expense of security'. She was able to offer no explanation for this difference.

In many studies, gender and kin relationship have been confounded. Studies have not always distinguished between mothers and fathers, but have included both as parents. Rogler and Hollingshead's (1965) study showed a more destructive impact on family organisation where men were caring for their wives. The fact that husbands in this Puerto Rican society were less willing to adopt elements of the wife's role may be an issue more concerned with gender or with race than with kinship. Similarly, it is not clear whether the reason that wives of depressed husbands showed a higher level of social isolation than did male carers is because they were married or because they were women (Fadden et al., 1987b). That women often found it upsetting to have to adopt traditional male roles, such as employment, even when these were performed competently, suggests that it was the gender role change which was particularly difficult.

However, none of these studies was set up specifically to examine any differential impact associated with gender. In addition, Kreisman and Joy (1974) noted that the majority of studies in their review focused on women's perceptions and attitudes as they relate to male patients. This has resulted in 'meagre knowledge' about the perceptions and expectations of males, and about the differential impact on the family of illness in men or women. This is true also of the main carer literature, though Parker's (1989) study of non-elderly spouse carers has explored some of the complexities of gender and caring, a subject also addressed by Ungerson (1987).

Other socio-demographic characteristics

Other socio-demographic variables investigated in this body of literature have been examined in correlational studies, and these, like those reported above in regard to kin relationship, age and gender, show no difference in strain for carers. Variables studied in this way include social class (Gibbons et al.; Thompson and Doll) and race and education (Thompson and Doll). Gubman and Tessler pointed out that 'caregiving obligations and options vary by social class', with American middle class families being more likely to use money as a resource and working class families more likely to use time, goods and physical space (1987, p.236). This is compatible with the point made above in relation to age and differential impact: that the overall impact may not differ with particular variables, because each age or class have particular stresses that are difficult for families to bear. This may explain why these findings, that socio-demographic variables are not associated with differential strain for carers, bear little relation to the evidence in the general carer literature.

These findings can also be contrasted with recent qualitative studies in this country that illustrate important differences in caring roles with regard to race (Cameron, Badger, Evers and Atkin, 1989).

These differences are unlikely to be amenable to quantitative measurement and analysis, as they are bound up with the deep-rooted preconceptions that white researchers have of the caring as of other situations. These preconceptions have meant that ethnocentric measures of stress and conceptualisations of health or of the family situation have been treated as universally applicable. More recently, discourse analysis has been used to demonstrate the ethnocentric assumptions that underlie disability (Atkin, 1989).

Some researchers, for instance Cheadle et al. (1978), have looked at the household composition of patients, though they do not always relate this to impact on the carer. Gibbons et al. (1984) reported that whether the carer lived alone with the patient, or together with other family members, there was no increased strain for the carer. In contrast, Crotty and Kulys (1986) found that strain was greatest for carers in larger, rather than smaller, households. It seems likely that from the point of view of the carer, both living alone with the dependant and with other family members offers advantages and disadvantages. Carers living in a smaller household may have fewer social contacts and a more restricted lifestyle, but may also have fewer sources of conflict and less responsibility for other family members. The evidence so far is inconclusive.

As with the kin relationship findings, it seems likely that the impact of caring differs for different sectors of society, but that this diversity is not always revealed by the overall assessments used in quantitative approaches. This, in conjunction with the fact that studies are based on only those families that have survived intact, may mean that we know about socio-demographic variables only for a particular sub-group of families. We can generalise to those families that cope with caring for someone with mental illness, but not to all families where mental illness occurs, to families from different social, racial and economic backgrounds, or to individual family members.

The previous four sections have been concerned with various socio-demographic characteristics of carers. Several issues can be drawn together at this point. The situation of spouse carers of people with mental illness is one which has received special attention, in contrast to the rest of the carer literature. However, many studies appear to confound gender issues with those of the spousal relationship. Moreover, the focus of these studies has generally been the patient rather than the carer. This means that the spouse carer is perceived as an adjunct to the patient's well-being rather than as of concern in his or her own right. Further, it is generally male patients who have been the focus, and women the spouse carers. This emphasis on the female carer/male patient may serve to mask the differential impact of caring on men and women. It underlines the point made by Finch (1987), Dalley (1987) and Ungerson (1987) that caring is often seen as an extension of women's roles. It also shows how there is a transferring of gendered notions into the process of research, constraining the definition of what is an appropriate area for investigation.

One further consideration concerns the measures used to assess strain in the carer. Briscoe (1982) and others have examined gender bias in measures of psychiatric distress. Many instruments which are in wide use include indicators which appear to produce a higher score for women than for men. In addition, cultural expectations may inhibit men from reporting emotional distress. There may be a consistent distortion of the outcome measure which results in women being assessed as showing more strain. A more appropriate approach to the issue of differential impact may be to assume a diversity of experience. It seems likely that, as research on race and informal care continues, more precise accounts of differential impact will be developed, as they have for gender.

Characteristics of the identified patient

Some studies have shown that personal characteristics of the dependent person do not affect the carer's experience (Seymour and Dawson, 1986; Thompson and Doll, 1982). Others have shown that there is a differential impact for families, but that this operates in a complex way:

> The high-risk indicators for being seen as a burden are lack of a confidant when present in combination with some of the following characteristics: being a woman, being young, being well educated, and living in a large household. (Crotty and Kulys, 1986, p.186)

One way of explaining this finding is to use gender as the basis for analysis. Certain types of behaviour (the more florid symptoms of schizophrenia, for instance) may be more easily tolerated in men than in women because society holds different expectations of men and women. A different set of expectations may be placed on young women who are well educated and still living in the parental home, as against young men in this situation. Findings need to be interpreted within the context of cultural expectations.

Associations between characteristics of the dependant and differential impact on the family are not straightforward and this may help to explain why evidence is sometimes contradictory. The notion that the caring situation is likely to be complex supports the inference made above that there are limitations to the usefulness of correlational studies as a means to understanding what life is like for carers. It may be more appropriate to adopt approaches that use more complex statistical techniques (Noh, 1985) or qualitative methods.

There is more agreement about the impact of the clinical status of the identified patient on the caring situation. Disturbed behaviour, current clinical characteristics and a more recent onset of psychiatric symptoms were particularly distressing to relatives interviewed by Gibbons et al. (1984). McCreadie et al. (1987) found that both social function and GHQ scores in relatives were associated with patients' clinical status as measured by the Present State Examination (PSE) though not as measured by four other clinical assessment measures. The neurotic symptoms of the patient mainly accounted for this correlation. The authors interpret this as demonstrating that while carers respond to anxiety in the dependant by themselves showing symptoms of anxiety, this is not the case for people caring for those with psychotic symptoms. Here, carers adapt to the situation, in that they show fewer psychiatric symptoms. Presumably, this adaptation implies either separation from or adjustment to the situation, although McCreadie implies adjustment only.

The relationship between clinical status of the identified patient and family well-being, though well established (Hirsch and Leff, 1975), is again complex. Platt and Hirsch (1981) reported that disturbed behaviour in patients caused greater distress for the family than either their social performance or disruption to household routine. Thompson and Doll (1982) found that carers were consistently and significantly upset while the dependant was exhibiting psychiatric symptoms. However, lack of current symptoms did not necessarily mean that carers were not distressed by the situation. The past, present and anticipated clinical status of former patients all aroused feelings of being trapped, overloaded and resentful, while recent admission to hospital was more likely to be associated with feelings of embarrassment. Fadden and her colleagues (1987b) found differences in the ways that different psychiatric symptoms among former patients affected carers. Florid symptoms of depressed spouses produced fewer emotional difficulties for carers than the negative and more persistent symptoms such as withdrawal or apathy. The authors point out that this may be tempered by bias in reporting, as few spouses were experiencing florid symptoms at time of interview and add that 'there is no doubt that relatives were upset at times of acute disturbance' (p.667).

Several studies have examined hospital admission and its impact on the carer. Crotty and Kulys (1986) found that there was no association between how recently the patient had been in hospital and its impact on the household member who offered most support. Seymour and Dawson (1986) monitored change before and after the discharge of a schizophrenic relative from hospital, and found deterioration in the quality of life for carers, particularly when carers were elderly and the patient had been ill for greater lengths of time. However, their exceptionally low response rate of 14 per cent raises questions about the generalisability of their findings.

There is no doubt that, over a long period of time, studies have shown that relatives caring for someone diagnosed as mentally ill have a higher level of psychiatric symptoms than the population as a whole. There is also strong evidence to show that, of all the aspects of the caring situation so far reported, it is the psychiatric status of the former patient which is most frequently associated with this family distress.

Social support

Just as there are aspects of the caring situation that exacerbate the impact on families, so are there aspects that may moderate it. Among these is the well-established role of effective social support in moderating the detrimental effects of life events (Brown and Harris, 1978) such as bereavement (Walker, MacBride and Vachon, 1977). Social support appears to be important in the caring situation also, for both carer and dependant. Crotty and Kulys (1986) found that when a schizophrenic patient had a confiding relationship and when relatives perceived this to be the case, there was decreased family burden. They linked this latter factor with an earlier study (citing Lowenthal, 1964) which reported lower hospital admission rates for elderly psychiatric patients with confidants.

This work is particularly important in the context of the widespread experience of disruption to social life of families reported above, and of investigations of the social life of schizophrenic patients. Sommer and Osmond (1984) noted that the presence of a schizophrenic member 'tends to isolate the family from the community', and in support of this cited Creer and Wing (1974), Doll (1976), and Pasamanick, Scarpetti and Dinitz (1967). They observed that the social isolation of patients that is apparent in hospital continues once the patient is discharged into the community. This is, they argued, a particular feature of schizophrenic illness, as ex-prisoners do not show this social isolation and therefore institutionalisation cannot be held responsible for this feature. Questions can be raised, however, about the validity of their choice of comparison group and about the fact that they explored neither causality nor possible links between stigma and concealment reported by Kreisman and Joy.

Despite such criticisms, it does appear that social isolation is both a feature of schizophrenia and a particularly distressing experience for relatives. If, as Crotty and Kulys have shown, better levels of social support serve to modify the burden carried by families, then interventions which reduce social isolation of either the former patient or their families may be particularly helpful.

Conclusion

There is mixed evidence about the differential impact of caring from studies of socio-demographic variables such as age, gender, class and race. It is clear that more basic research is needed with regard to these issues, but it is also apparent that, particularly with regard to race, there are fundamental preconceptions (that amount to misperceptions) that need adjusting. It seems likely that the diversity of the caring situation has produced a diversity of findings. Two issues do seem to be clear from the evidence so far available, however. The psychiatric status of the former patient, and effective social support for the carer and the person being cared for, both have definite effects on the families' reporting of the situation as more or less burdensome.

CHAPTER FOUR

Families and service provision

It is clear that carers of relatives with mental illness face considerable difficulties. It may therefore be surprising that a number of studies have shown that carers prefer their mentally ill relative to be living in the community where possible. They are generally willing to support their relative in order for them to do this. For instance, Johnstone et al. (1984) found in their study of the long-term impact of caring for schizophrenic patients that 27 of their 42 informants were satisfied with the patient's presence at home, and only six felt the patient should live elsewhere. Sixteen relatives reported the patient's clinical condition was satisfactory while five felt the clinical problems were so severe that they should be dealt with elsewhere. Johnstone and her co-workers concluded that care 'was provided by relatives who were in many cases frail, ageing, and coping only with great difficulty' (p.589). Despite the many problems arising from the patients' illness, these relatives rarely expressed a wish for the patient to return to hospital. Further, relatives find the task is manageable when support is available from services, and that it is facilitated when families and patients form part of the service planning (Hoult, 1986).

These findings can be compared with West et al.'s survey (1983, 1984 cited in Parker, 1985) of popular views of where services should be provided for different dependency groups. Just over 85 per cent of their respondents drawn from a general population thought that some form of community care was the most appropriate form of provision for non-elderly adults with a psychiatric disorder, although community care does not necessarily equate with family care. This has been seen in studies which traced former psychiatric patients now living in the community (Jones, Robinson and Golightly, 1986; Perring, Hunt, Parry and O'Connor, 1987).

Research on the effect of service provision on families with a mentally ill member has focused, as has much research on mental illness in the community, on the course of the illness in the community, on the individual diagnosed as mentally ill and, in particular, on how the course of the illness is affected by different ways of providing service. Only occasionally have studies recognised and sought to assess the impact of different treatment programmes in terms of family well-being. For mental illness, as for other forms of provision, it is even more rare for families to be asked for their own response to service provision.

All of this limits the relevance of the studies with regard to an understanding of the impact of service provision on carers. However, there are three broad areas that are relevant: the differential impact on families of traditional and community-based services; forms of service that aim to provide information to families on specific aspects of mental illness; and those few studies that have had as their primary focus families' attitudes to and experience of service provision.

The impact of formal support

Braun et al. (1981) reviewed 38 outcome studies of different programmes of care for psychiatric patients and recognised the importance of measuring the impact of these programmes on family members. Although several of the researchers mentioned in their review also noted this, few have pursued it. Evidence from studies that compare hospital- and community-based treatment is cited in only limited detail by Braun et al., and is contradictory with regard to impact on families. Two studies demonstrated that family burden was greater when service was provided only in the community. These were the studies conducted in Britain in the 1960s (Brown et al., 1966; Grad and Sainsbury, 1968). In contrast, a study by Washburn et al. (1976) showed that day treatment produced less distress and family burden than a traditional hospital stay. Hertz, Endicott and Spitzer and their co-workers (1976–1979); Pasamanick and colleagues (1967, 1974); Stein, Test and Marx (1975) and Test and Stein (1978) reported that different forms of, or alternatives to, hospital care produced no significant differences in the impact on families.

There are many possible reasons for these contradictory findings. Follow-up periods for the different studies vary from six months to five years, with the exception of that by Washburn et al. where no follow-up period is mentioned. Studies evaluate a variety of programmes that include day care, modified hospital care (day care and short-term care) and alternatives to hospital care. The studies are of differing designs – non-experimental (Brown et al.), controlled trial (Grad and Sainsbury) and randomised trial (the remaining four studies). They define 'families' in different ways, and it is not always specified whether these are co-resident with the former patient. Two studies were conducted in Britain (those of Brown and Grad and their colleagues) and the remainder in the United States. The interventions took place from the early 1960s to the late 1970s. The only study that reported that a non-traditional approach was better for families was that of Washburn et al. The findings of this study are limited because there appears to be no follow-up period, and the study was based on a highly selected sample, which reduces its generalisability.

Studies conducted after Braun et al.'s review include those of Test and Stein (1980), Hoult's (1986) replication of this in Australia, and Platt and Hirsch (1981). While attending to family well-being, these continue to emphasise outcome for the patient. The studies of Test and Hoult and their associates showed how intervention programmes could improve prognosis for patients for the lifetime of the programme, without detriment to the family. Test and Stein allocated families to either an experimental group or to a control group. Treatment for the experimental group was conducted entirely in the community. Treatment for the control group consisted of short-term hospitalisation plus after-care — in other words, a traditional approach. Families in the experimental group were not adversely affected in terms of disruption to the family when compared to the control group. The authors pointed to certain limitations of their study. They emphasised the difficulties of obtaining an adequate response rate for the follow-up interviews with families. Of 50 eligible families in each of the two groups, fewer than half responded at the two follow-up interviews. They also pointed to the absence of any measure for personal experience of distress.

Hoult and his colleagues replicated the intervention study in Australia (1984, 1986). They assigned 120 psychiatric patients to either an experimental or a control group. Intensive support from an interdisciplinary team was available at short notice (30 minutes) on a 24 hour, everyday basis. Relatives in general regarded the community-based treatment positively; this included about half of the relatives who were resident with a patient. One respondent reported appreciation at being able to share the load so that the patient, with the fear of hospital admission removed, was able to seek help more promptly and thus avoid more severe relapse. The experience of community treatment was particularly valuable for a group of 11 first-episode patients, only four of whom were admitted to hospital in the 12-month study period. This was in contrast to 11 of 12 first-episode patients in the control group who needed hospital admission. Clinical status of the experimental group was significantly better than that of the control group at 12 months. Hoult argues that for staff, who preferred the mode of working, for relatives and for patients, the intensive community programme was preferable.

These studies are important because they demonstrate that treatment programmes based entirely in the community, but in two different countries, can offer improved well-being to family members. Taken together, they show benefit both for families and their mentally ill relative. However, both studies reported that once the experimental intervention ceased, there was no carry-over benefit. Further, the level of intervention was much higher than that of treatment normally offered in the community.

Platt and Hirsch (1981) reported that in the short term there were no overall differences for families where patients had been randomly allocated to either brief or standard hospital care. This reproduced the findings of Hertz and co-workers in the 1970s. Measures were taken at points in time one month before, and two weeks and 14 weeks after hospital admission. These covered distress and various aspects of family life. Individual correlations showed more distress for families with patients allocated 'Brief Care' at two weeks with regard to the patient's 'slowness', but less distress with regard to impact on 'family performance in employment' compared to 'Standard Care' families. At 14 weeks, standard care families showed more distress with respect to their own social and leisure activities and the patient's personal neglect, but less distress than brief care families over the patient's over-dependence.

Intensive and long-term intervention from services in the community can ensure that families' quality of life is not impoverished beyond an unbearable level and can also provide a better quality of life for the former patient than life in hospital. Generalisations from this conclusion must be made with utmost caution. These studies are evaluations of service provision that has been constructed for research purposes. They were not situations with normal levels of service provision. Research sampling methods have often over-estimated the level of service, and intervention studies have deliberately increased service provision. It is likely that the levels of formal support normally available to families are considerably lower than those evaluated in research projects, and certainly unlikely to be of the same order as the provision evaluated in intervention studies such as Hoult's. In addition, studies with a range of follow-up periods demonstrate that any benefits are unlikely to continue once the intensive programme of care has ended. It is inappropriate to extrapolate directly from findings that show that community-based care is superior without examining the level and long term effects of that care.

Families' knowledge about the situation

The need for knowledge and information about the situation in which carers find themselves has been widely reported and emphasised, both in the literature under review here (Hatfield, 1979) and in the carer literature (Glendinning, 1983; Levin, Sinclair and Gorbach, 1983). Atkinson (1986), however, found that relatives provided and wide range of responses to questions about their situation, and concluded that the need for information was less salient than needs likely to be met by other service provision:

> The two problems which the greatest number of relatives mentioned were 'the future' and 'getting help when it's needed'. These were followed by the social problems of the patient, family friction and supervision. The three areas of help which relatives reported wanting most were: day care of some kind; changes in 'the professional approach'; direct help for relatives.
> (Atkinson, 1986, p.175)

As these problems are potentially affected through appropriate information-giving, Atkinson's conclusions are not necessarily incompatible with other work on providing information to families.

Most of the studies that have been reported have assessed the impact of knowledge about schizophrenia on families' ability to cope with mental illness. One important way in which information has been conveyed to families is through psychoeducation. This is a systematic and formalised way of providing families with information about the origins, course and experience of mental illness. This may take place in a variety of ways including family support groups, the provision of written material and family therapy. A significant amount of psychoeducation is now based on the influential theory of 'expressed emotion'. Here, a number of studies have shown prognosis is unfavourable in families where high levels of hostile or critical comment occur (the studies of Brown and Falloon and their colleagues, 1962, 1972 and 1982; see Kuipers, 1979, for a review of research on expressed emotion). Two recent studies have examined the role of expressed emotion in a setting that emphasises relatives' groups and counselling (Leff, Berkowitz, Shavit, Strachan, Glass and Vaughn, 1989; MacCarthy, Kuipers, Hurry, Harper and LeSage, 1989a). Both studies recommend relatives' groups as effective, but while Leff and colleagues stress the role of expressed emotion,

MacCarthy et al. see the opportunity for relatives of being able to share some of their 'pent-up' feelings as an appropriate focus for intervention.

Barrowclough and Tarrier and their colleagues (1987, 1989) evaluated the role of psychoeducation in outcome for patients. They found that a substantial number of relatives were unlikely to modify their lay model of schizophrenia, particularly where the patient had a relatively long history of illness. Barrowclough and his colleagues developed the Knowledge about Schizophrenia Interview (KASI) together with an information booklet designed to be incorporated into an education programme based on theories of expressed emotion. KASI can be used to identify relatives whose attitudes may prove detrimental to the future course of the illness and who may therefore need extra advice and support. The researchers concluded that it is possible to run brief educational programmes with families which would lead to actions that will assist in the patients' recovery both in the short and in the longer term. Their study is within the tradition of focusing on patient, rather than on family well-being and it provides no indication of whether families themselves benefit from increased information.

There have also been studies concerned with psychoeducation outside this tradition. For instance, Ferris and Marshall (1987) described an educational project for families of chronically ill people within the 'nonblaming-stance' (citing Jung, Spaniol and Anthony, 1983). Here, an attitude is adopted by professional workers which explicitly avoids attributing blame to the family for either the origins or lack of improvement of mental illness. Ferris and Marshall proposed that education about the nature and management of schizophrenia, about effective communication, and about problem-solving skills was particularly helpful to families. While stressing that this is not an evaluation, they pointed out a number of activities that can help families. These include educational workshops and seminars attended by families, clients and professionals, establishing a thrift shop which offers sheltered employment for clients, and developing an advocacy role to improve state facilities. They note that there is also an enhancement of families' lifestyle from the improved and increased social contact associated with these activities. The question must be posed, then, as to whether the improved family situation was associated with increased information or with increased social contact. It seems likely that improved contact with service providers is an integral aspect of educational programmes: only an appropriately designed study would disentangle the relative contributions of improved information, improved social support and closer and more harmonious contact with professional workers.

There has been a trend towards the publication of books such as those by Anderson, Reiss and Hogarty (1986) or Atkinson (1986) which offer advice to practitioners and families on the management of schizophrenia in a family setting. Anderson et al. offer a model treatment programme and illustrate its application. They emphasis the need for professional workers and families to work as allies in reducing the stress experienced when mentally ill people live with families, and their programme of psychoeducation provides a planned and gradual way of achieving this. This programme is reviewed, together with other forms of aftercare for schizophrenics living at home, by Iodice and Wodarski (1987).

One finding that is unexpected in the context of this body of work on the beneficial role of information for families was reported by Namyslowska (1986). She found that people who were 'better informed about the illness are coping with its stress much less efficiently' (p.403). She proposed that use of a defence mechanism such as denial may be the most adaptive way of with chronic stress. She pointed out that this is in conflict with one view in systems theory which states that additional information is vital for a system under threat (such as a family) to be able to retain its structure.

This finding is atypical, and psychoeducation appears to be an increasingly important element in service provision. However, it was originally introduced in order to improve the situation for the dependent person, and this continues to be its primary focus. It should be seen as only one element in a package of provision. A service that aims to promote family well-being needs to emphasis other aspects of service provision that remain important to families, as well as psychoeducation.

Evaluating provision from the perspective of carers

It is important to remember that services have been primarily designed to meet the needs of the identified patient, although they will often benefit carers either directly or indirectly. This off-centre relationship is evident across the field of carer support (Twigg, Atkin and Perring, 1990). Comments from carers reflect this orientation in service provision. Several studies have canvassed carers for their views about their experience of existing services. Carers have also been asked about services which they might wish to receive, and some studies have asked carers for their opinions about what might be an 'ideal provision' (Perring, Hunt, Parry and O'Connor, 1987).

Studies have pointed to the generally low quality and quantity of carers' contact with services, both where respondents are drawn from relatives already in contact with some form of service provision (Creer 1975) and from a more general sample (Johnstone et al. 1984; Perring et al., 1987). Most of Creer's and Perring et al.'s respondents reported instances of contact with one especially helpful worker, though many voiced specific criticisms of the level of involvement by services. Johnstone and her co-workers (1984) found in their follow-up study that 51 of 66 families had no contact with a social worker, and that the greatest levels of distress were found among patients and their families receiving no social or medical attention.

Relatives have voiced a number of concerns about the quality of provision. Poor long-term involvement with professional workers is a particularly common criticism (Creer, 1975; Johnstone et al., 1984). This takes several forms such as frequent staff changes and the lack of opportunity for long-term contact with a constant figure who knows the patient's case (Johnstone et al.), ignoring parents' concerns until a crisis point is reached and compulsory hospital admission occurs (Creer; Creer, Sturt and Wykes, 1982), and lack of advice on the patient's return home from hospital (Creer). A second major theme is the attitude displayed by professional workers who were seen as unsympathetic to carers' difficulties (Creer). They failed to recognize family burden (Johnstone et al.), and poor communication between relatives and workers was experienced in the 'politely cool reception' accorded to relatives (Creer, Sturt and Wykes, p.37). Support from service providers also came from unanticipated sources, such as the police; for instance, when the dependant's behaviour was so disturbed that compulsory hospital admission became necessary (Perring et al., 1987). In this study, relatives did not report any one single form of service provision as being particularly helpful; they were more likely to name one individual from among the range of workers with whom they were in contact.

Other studies, such as those by McCreadie and his co-workers (1987) and MacCarthy et al. (1989a), have pointed out the importance of the timing of service involvement with families. This should begin as soon as the patient first enters hospital or early in the 'patient's career', and is for the well-being of both patient and family. The importance of the duration of service involvement has been demonstrated by the intervention studies reported earlier in this paper (Hoult, 1986; Test and Stein, 1980) which report that any benefits are lost once the intervention period ends. Permanent and appropriately-timed community support is therefore essential.

Overall, Creer reported that although one quarter of her respondents were satisfied with services, nearly one third were very dissatisfied.

It will be remembered that her respondents included a high proportion of relatives in contact with services, and may therefore be a special sample. While her study provides a clear commentary on those services which are received, it is likely to under-report the general experience of service receipt. In particular, her study does not represent the views of those who have withdrawn from service provision, possibly because of dissatisfaction with the service.

One important aspect of service that has been singled out for comment is co-operation between relatives and professional workers. There is a consensus among studies reviewed here that close co-operation is essential for the well-being of patient and relative alike (Hatfield, 1979; Iodice and Wodarski, 1987; Thompson and Doll, 1982). Studies that have assessed the nature of the relationship between relatives and professional workers have rarely shown that this co-operation is satisfactory from the relatives' point of view.

Other gaps in service provision have also been identified by asking respondents directly. Creer pointed to problems of access to suitable service at the onset of a first episode of schizophrenia. Creer's relatives also wanted day care, respite breaks and greater communication with professional staff. Northouse (1980) has commented on the absence of routine pathways to link families to sources of relief. Johnstone found that relatives believed that service providers lost interest in patients over time when they did not become well. Additional support at times of crisis was mentioned by relatives in the study by Perring et al. Fadden (1987b) and her co-workers, who asked similar questions of relatives of depressed patients, reported that relatives wanted information, consultation over treatment and earlier admission to hospital. All of these appear to be requesting closer contact with existing services. At different stages in the course of mental illness, then, inadequate services have been identified by carers themselves. Onset, times of crisis, periods of respite between crises and the need for long-term support, especially for those who show no improvement, are all situations which require different types of support for carers.

We must also devote some attention to the concept of unreported need. This is a problematic and contested concept, and Creer and Wing (1974) have succinctly pointed to processes that may contribute to low expectations, low demands and unmet needs:

> So certain characteristics of relatives can result in their needs being left unmet. They do not always see that they have a need. If they do perceive this, they may feel they have no right to ask for help or may not know that there are services intended to meet their needs. (Creer and Wing, 1974).

In addition, some of the reasons why relatives hold low expectations about formal support concern service provision itself. It is the nature of many services to be demand-led and non-intrusive, and to assume that those in need will ask for services. However, services which respond to crisis, rather than to prevention or maintenance, may not be the most appropriate form of service for carers with responsibilities for long-term care. Creer and Wing found that even 'articulate and knowledgeable' relatives did not always have their needs met by such a service.

Low expectation can be detected by discrepancies in statistics. Fadden et al. (1987a) citing Hoenig and Hamilton (1966, 1969), commented that of relatives who felt that no more could be done for them, three quarters experienced objective burden and half reported subjective burden. However, fewer than one tenth complained about services. An empirical investigation of the perspectives held by former psychiatric patients, their relatives and professional workers has revealed a number of differences in the perception of need:

> Thus, when relatives perceive budgeting as an area of need not recognised by former patients, or when professional workers point to inadequacies in a social network with which former patients express satisfaction, sites of possible unreported need can be identified. (Perring, forthcoming).

Other research teams have attempted to assess levels of unmet need with regard to service provision (Creer et al., 1982; MacCarthy, LeSage, Brewin, Brugha, Mangen and Wing, 1989b). Creer and her colleagues reported that two thirds of their 52 interviewees wanted some change to their present service, and that one third of relatives had at least one unmet need. The most common request was for practical help such as financial advice. Involvement in planning a treatment programme, information about managing difficult behaviour, breaks from caring and emotional support were other needs frequently unmet by current services MacCarthy and her colleagues used Brewin and Wing's *Needs for Care Assessment* to identify unmet needs among relatives. They found that relatives expressed little dissatisfaction with services and were mostly resigned to their situation, despite a large number of unmet needs. The highest rate of under-provision was with regard to emotional burden, which was widespread among the relatives. MacCarthy et al. recommend that the assessment of unmet need be included as part of routine clinical practice 'in order to ensure that they [the relatives] are adequately supported in the key role they play in the provision of community care'. In some studies, high levels of unmet need have been identified. Holden and Lewine (1982) suggest that these levels may under-report unmet need, given the characteristics of the people who participated in their study.

Several reasons for such widespread unmet need have been suggested. These include under-reporting of need (Creer and Wing, 1974), low expectation among respondents (Fadden et al., 1987a), inadequate assessment (Creer, Sturt and Wykes, 1982), professional workers assuming that tolerance among families implies no need for enhanced services (Fadden et al., 1987a), and the difficulties of providing a service to ease emotional burden (MacCarthy et al., 1989b).

The difficulties facing families of people who are mentally ill are diverse and numerous and it may be difficult to construct a package of services to match their needs. Creer and Wing (1974) have pointed out that professionals target their services at the patient, and that no professional group exists to offer support to relatives in their own right. Even studies aimed at improving services to relatives use well-being of the patient as an argument for doing so (Katschnig and Konieczna, 1989). Researchers, too, have often focused on patient, rather than family, well-being. Despite this lack of attention, a number of service-related factors have been shown to reduce the emotional distress of carers and the family disturbance which may be experienced as a result of caring at home for someone with mental illness. These include close contact with service providers (Birchwood and Smith, 1987; Hoult, 1986; Test and Stein, 1980); the provision of information and advice to relatives (Barrowclough et al., 1987); and day care provision (McCreadie et al., 1987). MacCarthy et al. (1989b) proposed that such services should be provided in flexible ways, and saw this as particularly important because of the long-term nature of family burden. Although these studies have often focused on the effect of provision of service for the dependent person, it can be concluded that those families which are intact cope with their caring tasks with comparatively few complaints, despite an absence of services.

One particular point to note is that no study so far reported has included information from families after care has ended. The purpose of service provision in relation to the ending of care is controversial, since the ending of care is likely to raise the issue of conflicting interests between carer and dependant. Some services may have the prevention of care breakdown as an explicit aim, while others may promote independent living as an appropriate goal for carer and dependant. This is likely to be related to service providers' views of carers as resources, co-workers or co-clients (Twigg, 1989).

Conclusion

There is an inevitable tension between meeting the needs of the carer and the needs of the dependant, and this poses difficulties for providing a balanced service. Appropriate service provision is less likely to be available when the issue of unreported need is neglected, as in this situation it will be particularly difficult to ensure a balance in provision. It is difficult to maintain a focus on the needs of relatives and carers when the needs of patients are so clearly visible. This tendency is compounded when services are structured to focus on an identified patient or client and to regard families as a backdrop which may be contributing to the psychiatric ill-health of that patient.

The ability of families to cope against a background of inadequate formal support does not mean that services to families need no improvement. The issues of unreported need, the continuing evidence that care by the family is associated with various indicators of stress, and criticisms that families make of their experience with professional workers all underline the fact that some effective intervention for families with a mentally ill member is essential, for the benefit of family and identified patient alike.

CHAPTER FIVE

Where we are now

The purpose of this discussion paper has been twofold: to review such literature as is relevant to an understanding of the informal care of people diagnosed as mentally ill; and to begin to explore possible relationships between findings from the psychological and psychiatric literature on the one hand, and those from the work on informal care on the other. We are now in a position to develop our understanding of informal care in the light of the two bodies of research. We can begin by considering a few examples of different caring situations. These are drawn from four main areas: physical tasks and responsibility, restrictedness in family and social life, emotional distress and other less easily measured aspects of the situation, and service provision. We then move on to identify some of the gaps in understanding that may be addressed by future research.

Comparison with other carers

Much work on informal care has been concerned with the tasks of personal care and physical disability. This has had a profound influence on notions of what constitutes informal care. There are also caring situations, one of which is caring for someone diagnosed as mentally ill, where tasks of personal care are not the major feature of the situation. Responsibility and supervision can be prominent features of many caring situations, although the precise nature of this responsibility and supervision varies. Carers of people with learning difficulties are likely to have exercised considerable responsibility since the dependant's birth. This contrasts with the situation of carers of people with Alzheimer's Disease, who have taken on such responsibility at a later stage in the life of the dependent person. The responsibility exercised on behalf of someone who suffers from a degenerative disease is different from the responsibility necessary as a result of a mental impairment. With regard to mental illness, the responsibility is less clearly defined and sometimes only assumed periodically. This periodic quality is experienced by other categories of carer, for example, those caring for someone with multiple sclerosis or rheumatoid arthritis, but here responsibility is combined with physical care. In the case of mental illness, this defining feature tends to be absent and this may in the past have contributed to the exclusion of this category from the main carer literature.

Restriction of social life and leisure activities and disruption to family life are commonly reported in both sets of literature. Social life for all categories of carers has been shown to be severely restricted, and demonstrated throughout the literature to be highly distressing to those concerned. The reasons for restrictedness, however, vary with the impairment of the dependant and with characteristics (such as age, gender, race, health) of the carer. Thus, while carers of people who have been diagnosed as mentally ill may feel ashamed or embarrassed by the public behaviour of their dependant, carers of physically disabled people may face problems relating to the absence of appropriate physical access to public facilities. Both situations will limit carers' participation in 'normal' public life.

Social support, from both inside and outside the immediate family, has been shown to be difficult to obtain in a caring situation. In addition, the dependant may no longer be able to offer the same support as formerly. The notion of reciprocity appears to be central to an understanding of why carers find it difficult to make demands of family, neighbours or acquaintances. This appears to apply in both bodies of research. Disruption to other aspects of family life, such as employment and financial circumstances, have not been studied comprehensively enough to permit comparison with the situation of other carers. From Glendinning's (1989) work, it seems likely that the situation with regard to these aspects is complex, and this is an area where more basic research is needed.

Research reviewed here shows that carers commonly report the less easily measured aspects that relate to meaning and interpretation as more distressing than those that are clearer cut and therefore more easily measured. Some of these aspects, such as concerns that relate to bizarre behaviour or to loss of the person, are seen in several other caring situations. Coping with difficult behaviour, one of the aspects reported as particularly demanding by this group of carers, is also experienced by those caring for elderly people with senile dementia and for people with challenging behaviour. In particular, this may involve coping with suicide attempts and with violence. It is possible that in any of these caring situations, the family will have police or probation contact as a result of their relative's criminal or semi-criminal activity.

Abrupt change in the needs of a dependent person may arise because of a stroke, an accident, the onset of an incapacitating physical disease or the onset of mental illness. This change is likely to lead to extreme distress about the loss of the person, and about changes in responsibility and supervision of financial, medical and behavioural aspects of the dependant's life. Other aspects that are associated with particular emotional distress for carers, such as concern for the future, are also reported by carers of many different dependency groups. The particular aspect of the future that presents most emotional distress is, however, likely to vary with the particular situation. Most elderly carers, for instance, are likely to voice anxieties about the future well-being of their dependent offspring. Carers of people with mental illness are distressed by feeling stigmatised and ashamed by their situation. This distress is also reported by carers of other groups of people, such as those with learning difficulties or with HIV or AIDS (Miller, 1987).

In addition to the caring situation in the home, the review has also included the experience of carers with service providers. It might appear that this is one aspect of the situation that is unique to carers of people diagnosed as mentally ill, given possible links between dominant theories about mental illness and a stance among many professional workers that either explicitly or implicitly blames the carer for contributing to the origins or course of the diagnosed illness. This could be used to account for the exclusion of the carer from discussions about appropriate forms of care, or in comments from staff which cause distress to carers. This interpretation is likely to be an over-simplification of the situation, for difficulties are experienced by many carers with regard to their contact with services, even when the disease or disability is one that is not traditionally associated with theories that adopt a 'blaming' stance towards carers.

Remaining questions

This review has pointed to several sets of issues concerning informal care that warrant research attention. We have outlined one such issue above: namely, the need for a detailed comparison of the situation of those caring for mentally ill people with that of other carers. In addition, there are empirical and conceptual issues to be addressed.

Some possible refinements to the use of quantitative methods have been identified in the course of this review. Platt (1985) pointed to the need to identify the precise onset of any family disturbance, and to distinguish between the occurrence of any disturbance and the degree to which carers may attribute this to their dependant. He stressed that emotional responses can be reliably ascertained only from the informant concerned and not on behalf of another household member, and that in commenting on family or household disruption it is essential to identify the source of such information. Platt's typology is very comprehensive in identifying the various elements of the caring situation, and could be used to provide the basis of comparable, rather than idiosyncratic, measures of the caring situation. The technique of Creer and Wing and their colleagues, who sought information on actual events occurring within the month prior to interview, has the advantage of providing material that can be accurately recalled and that can offer instances of 'objective burden'. These instances can then be used as bases for an assessment of emotional response.

Other methodological improvements can be suggested. It is important to be certain that such distress as does occur in this situation is related to the presence of mental illness and is not merely a normal feature of family life. This requires either more studies that include control or comparison groups together with the research group, or more comparative work with the literature on family life. Many families do not survive intact when mental illness occurs and the experience of such families appears to be unresearched. Their experience may be particularly valuable in understanding the circumstances surrounding the ending of care. Similarly, attention to the start of the caring role and shifts in responsibility, and hence of family role, may elucidate differences in the task of caring for someone with mental illness as compared with other forms of caring. Comparatively few studies have investigated situations where mental illness other than schizophrenia has been diagnosed, and no study so far has addressed the periodic and fluctuating nature of many forms of mental distress and the impact this has on the carer or the family. The tendency of this body of literature to investigate the family as a whole fails to address the issue of considerable unanticipated responsibility falling consistently to one particular carer. Further, the family situation is assumed to be homogeneous, when in reality it may encompass spousal, sibling, or parental, as well as non-kin, relationships. Within these relationships, gender and age also have to be considered. This links with a second major area where more research is needed – the further theoretical development of informal care.

Addressing some of these issues will meet some of the substantive inadequacies that exist, such as those that concern the situation of people diagnosed as depressed, and the tendency to focus on the dependant, as a patient, rather than on the carer. Empirical research about other aspects of the caring situation is also needed. The relationship between the impact of caring on family disruption and the emotional distress experienced by carers is far from clear. It is possible that one carer may tolerate or cope with a situation which a second carer finds intolerable. It may be useful to include general models of coping with stress, as Avison and Speechley (1987) and Titterton (1989) propose, to address this aspect of informal care and personal welfare. This may provide an answer to the question of why it is that one carer is able to shrug off complaints from neighbours about loud noise, while another may feel profoundly disturbed. This will add depth at the psychological level to an understanding of the caring situation, and would introduce new approaches to meet some of the other points already raised. At the same time, such an approach would complement the understanding to be gained from, for instance, an analysis that is based on constraints at the structural level.

Although disruption to family life has been extensively documented, there is a less clear understanding of what makes caring easier for some people than for others. It seems unlikely that quantitative methods, such as those used in most of the studies reported here, will contribute to this understanding. For instance, race is one aspect of the situation that is increasingly recognised as contributing to a differential impact for carers (Atkin, Cameron, Evers and Badger, 1989). The integration of this work, together with research on race and mental illness, with the mainstream work on informal care will highlight some of the underlying assumptions in the field, such as the ethnocentrism of much of the work that is by white researchers and about white people. The differential impact of care is an additional area where more detailed work is required.

It is important to recognise that the above refinements relate principally to research that is conducted within a quantitative tradition, and that there are other ways in which informal care can be investigated. There is a need for a greater emphasis on process, understanding and meaning rather than simply on outcome. Work is needed at the conceptual level since, until now, the informal care of those diagnosed as mentally ill has mainly been seen as burden for families. There is little recognition of the possibility that carers may perceive the role in different terms, of the need to move away from the concept of burden as it is used in the body of work reviewed here, or of the need to refer to individual carers, rather than to families. The term burden is misleading in certain ways. Many relatives wish to care for their dependants, and it is not clear whether they see this task as a burden. Creer and Wing have suggested the use of 'support' as a more appropriate word, and the word 'supporter' is now more widely used than formerly. The term implies, however, a continuing focus on the patient, as someone who is being 'supported', and the relegation of the carer to a secondary role.

Secondly, the significance of the relationship between carer and cared-for person has not been fully considered. As Twigg (1989) has pointed out, carers are in an ambiguous and ill-defined position. While we are arguing that carers should be seen in their own right and that future work should address the previous imbalance of focus, it is also important to realise that carers are often significant to service providers and policy makers only because of their relationship with the cared-for person. This relationship may give rise to a potential conflict of interest between carer and cared-for person over compulsory outpatient treatment, for instance (Mulvey, Geller and Roth, 1987). This has only rarely been addressed empirically (Perring, forthcoming), but can also be examined at a conceptual level where responsibility, shifts in responsibility and how these relate to individual rights can be explored. The issue of rights tends to be clearer for people with learning difficulties, where responsibility appears to be constant, than for people diagnosed as mentally ill, where a sense of responsibility is more likely to fluctuate with episodes of distress. Both of these examples are in sharp contrast with the success of advocacy movements among those with physical impairment (e.g. war veterans in the US) that have campaigned for access to public facilities.

Conclusion

We have reviewed studies from the psychological and psychiatric literature and provided a detailed description of what life is like for those caring for someone diagnosed as mentally ill. We have also begun to integrate this work with the carer literature and, in doing so, have highlighted some areas where additional research is needed. Many aspects of the caring situation are common to both sets of circumstances. Despite some differences, we would argue that it is entirely appropriate to apply the concept of informal care to the situation of people diagnosed as mentally ill. We would further argue that doing so will clarify and enrich our understanding of informal care.

Bibliography

ANDERSON, C. M., REISS, D. N. and HOGARTY, G.E. (1986) *Schizophrenia and the Family: A Practitioner's Guide to Psychoeducation and Management*. New York: Guildford Press.

ARMSTRONG, D. (1983) *The Political Anatomy of the Body*. Cambridge: University of Cambridge Press.

ATKIN, K. (1989) 'Disability and black minorities: the problems of humanist discourse.' Social Policy Research Unit, University of York.

ATKIN, K. CAMERON, E., EVERS, H. and BADGER, F. (1989) *Black Perspectives on Health: A Conceptual Appraisal*. Birmingham: Health Service Research Centre, University of Birmingham.

ATKINSON, S. M. (1986) *Schizophrenia at Home: A Guide to Helping the Family*. New York: New York University Press.

AVISON, W. R. and SPEECHLEY, K. N. (1987) 'The discharged psychiatric patient: a review of social, social-psychological and psychiatric correlates of outcome.' *American Journal of Psychiatry*, 144 (1), pp 10–18.

BARROWCLOUGH, C. and TARRIER, N. (1984) 'Psychosocial interventions with families and their effects on the course of schizophrenia: a review.' *Psychological Medicine*, 14, pp 629–642.

BARROWCLOUGH, C., TARRIER, N., WATTS, S., VAUGHN, C., BAMRAH, J. S. and FREEMAN, H. L. (1987) 'Assessing the functional value of relatives' knowledge about schizophrenia: a preliminary report.' *British Journal of Psychiatry*, 151, (July), pp 1–8.

BIRCHWOOD, M. and SMITH, J. (1987) 'Schizophrenia and the Family.' In J. Orford (ed), *Coping with Disorder in the Family*. London: Croom Helm.

BRADSHAW, J. (1972) 'A Taxonomy of Social Need.' In G. McLachlan (ed), *Problems and Progress in Medical Care*. London: Oxford University Press.

BRAUN, P., KOCHANSKY, G., SHAPIRO, R., GREENBERG, S., GOUDEMAN, J. E., JOHNSON, S. and SHORE, M. F. (1981) 'Overview: deinstitutionalization of psychiatric patients: a critical review of outcome studies.' *American Journal of Psychiatry*, 13, pp 736–749.

BRISCOE, M. (1982) 'Sex differences in psychological well-being.' *Psychological Medicine*, 12, Monograph Supplement 1.

BROMET, E. J., ED, V. and MAY, S. (1984) 'Family environments of depressed outpatients.' *Acta Psychiatrica Scandinavica*, 13, pp 197–200.

BROWN, G. W., BIRLEY, J. L. T. and WING, J. K. (1972) 'The influence of family life on the course of schizophrenic disorders: a replication.' *British Journal of Psychiatry*, 13, pp 241–58.

BROWN, G. W. and HARRIS, T. O. (1978) *Social Origins of Depression: A Study of Psychiatric Disorder in Women*. London: Tavistock Publications.

BROWN, G. W., MONCK, E. M., CARSTAIRS, G. M. and WING, J. K. (1962) 'Influence of family life on the course of schizophrenic illness.' *British Journal of Preventive and Social Medicine*, 16, pp 55–68

CAMERON, E., BADGER, F., EVERS, H. and ATKIN, K. (1989) 'Black old women and health carers.' In M. Jefferys (ed) *Growing Old in the Twentieth Century*. London: Routledge.

CHEADLE, A. J., FREEMAN, H. L. and KORER, J. (1978) 'Chronic schizophrenic patients in the community.' *British Journal of Psychiatry*, 13, pp 221–7.

CHESLER, P. (1972) *Women and Madness*. New York: Doubleday.

CLAUSEN, J. A. and YARROW, M. R. (1955) 'The impact of mental illness on the family.' *Journal of Social Issues*, 11 (4) pp 6–11.

CREER, C. (1975) 'Living with schizophrenia.' *Social Work Today*, 6, pp 2–7.

CREER, C. and WING, J. K. (1974) *Schizophrenia at Home*. Surbiton: National Schizophrenia Fellowship.

CREER, C., STURT, E. and WYKES, T. (1982) 'The role of relatives.' In J. K. Wing (ed), 'Long-term community care experience in a London borough.' *Psychological Medicine*, 12, Monograph Supplement 2, pp 29–39.

CROTTY, P. and KULYS, R. (1986) 'Are schizophrenics a burden to their families? Significant others' views.' *Health and Social Work*, 11 (3), pp 173–188.

DALLEY, G. (1984) 'Ideologies of care: a feminist contribution to the debate.' *Critical Social Policy*, 3, (8, No.2), pp 72–81.

DEASY, L. C. and QUINN, O. W. (1955) 'The wife of the mental patient and the hospital psychiatrist.' *Journal of Social Issues*, 11, pp 49–60.

DH/DSS/WELSH OFFICE/SCOTTISH OFFICE (1989) *Caring for People: Community Care in the Next Decade and Beyond*. Cm 849, London: HMSO.

DOLL, W. (1976) 'Family coping with the mentally ill: an unanticipated problem of deinstitutionalization.' *Hostital and Community Psychiatry*, 23, pp 183–85.

FADDEN, G., BEBBINGTON, P. and KUIPERS, L. (1987a) 'The burden of care: the impact of functional psychiatric illness on the patient's family.' *British Journal of Psychiatry*, 150, pp 285–292.

FADDEN, G., BEBBINGTON, P. and KUIPERS, L. (1987b) 'Caring and its burdens: a study of relatives of depressed patients.' *British Journal of Psychiatry*, 150, pp 660–667.

FALLOON, I. R. H., BOYD, J. L., McGILL, G. W., RAZANI, J., MOOS, H. B. and GILDERMAN, A. M. (1982) 'Family management in the prevention of exacerbations of schizophrenia: a controlled study.' *New England Journal of Medicine*, 306, pp 437–40.

FERRIS, P. A. and MARSHALL, C. A. (1987) 'A model project for families of the chronically mentally ill.' *Social Work*, 32, pp 110–114.

FINCH, J. (1984) 'Community care: developing non-sexist alternatives.' *Critical Social Policy*, 9, (3 No.2), pp 6–18.

FINCH, J. (1989) *Family Obligations and Social Change*. Cambridge: Polity Press.

GIBBONS, J. S., HORN, S. M., POWELL, J. M. and GIBBONS, J. L. (1984) 'Schizophrenic patients and their families: a survey in a psychiatric service based on a DGH unit.' *British Journal of Psychiatry*, 144, pp 70–77.

GILHOOLY, M. L. M. (1984) 'The impact of care-giving on care-givers: factors associated with the psychological well-being of people supporting a dementing relative in the community.' *British Journal of Medical Psychology*, 57, pp 35–44.

GLENDINNING, C. (1983) *Unshared Care*. London: Routledge and Kegan Paul.

GLENDINNING, C. (1989) *The Financial Needs and Circumstances of Informal Carers: Final Report*. York: Social Policy Research Unit, University of York.

GRAD, J. and SAINSBURY, P. (1963) 'Mental illness and the family.' *Lancet*, i, pp 544–547.

GRAD, J. and SAINSBURY, P. (1968) 'The effects that patients have on their families in a community—care and a control psychiatric service: a two year follow-up.' *British Journal of Psychiatry*, 114, pp 265–278.

GRIFFITHS, R. (1987) *Community Care: An Agenda for Action*. London: HMSO.

GUBMAN, G. D. and TESSLER, R. C. (1987) 'The impact of mental illness on families' concepts and priorities.' *Journal of Family Issues*, 8, (2 June), pp 226–245.

HARDING, C. M., BROOKS, G. W. ASHIKAGA, T., STRAUSS, J. and BREIER, A. (1987) 'The Vermont longitudinal study of persons with severe mental illness, II: long-term outcome of subjects who retrospectively met DSM-III criteria for schizophrenia.' *American Journal of Psychiatry*, 144 (6), pp 727–735.

HATFIELD, A. B. (1979) 'The family as partners in the treatment of mental illness.' *Hospital and Community Psychiatry*, 30 (5), pp 338–340.

HATFIELD, A. B. and LEFLEY, H. P. (eds) (1987) *Families of the Mentally Ill: Coping and Adaptation*. London: Guildford Press.

HAWKS, D. (1975) 'Community care: an analysis of assumptions.' *British Journal of Psychiatry*, 127, pp 276–285.

HERTZ, M. I., ENDICOTT, J. and SPITZER, R. L. (1976) 'Brief versus standard hospitalization: the families.' *American Journal of Psychiatry*, 133 (7), pp 795–801.

HERTZ, M. I., ENDICOTT, J. and GIBBON, M. (1979) 'Brief hospitalization: two year follow-up.' *Archives of General Psychiatry*, 130, pp 701–705.

HIRSCH, S. R. and LEFF, J. P. (1975) *Abnormalities in Parents of Schizophrenics*. London: Oxford University Press.

HIRSCH, S. R., PLATT, S. D., KNIGHTS, A. and WEYMAN, A. (1979) 'Shortening hospital stay for psychiatric care: effect in patients and their families.' *British Medical Journal*, i, pp 442–446.

HOENIG, J. and HAMILTON, M. W. (1966) 'The schizophrenic patient in the community and his effect on the household.' *International Journal of Social Psychiatry*, 12, pp 165–176.

HOLDEN, D. F. and LEWINE, R. J. (1982) 'How families evaluate mental health professionals, resources, and effects of illness.' *Schizophrenia Bulletin*, 8 (4), pp 626–633.

HOULT, J. (1986) 'Community care of the acutely mentally ill.' *British Journal of Psychiatry*, 149, pp 137–144.

HOULT, J. and REYNOLDS, I. (1984) 'Schizophrenia: a comparative trial of community oriented and hospital oriented psychiatric care. *Acta Psychiatrica Scandinavica*, 69, pp 359–372.

INEICHEN, B. (1989) 'Afro-Caribbeans and the incidence of schizophrenia: a review.' *New Community*, 15 (3), pp 335–341.

IODICE, J. D. and WODARSKI, J. S. (1987) 'Aftercare treatment for schizophrenics living at home.' *Social Work*, 32 (2), pp 122–128.

JOHNSTONE, E. C., OWENS, D. G. C., GOLD, A., CROW, T. J. and MACMILLAN, J. F. (1984) 'Schizophrenic patients discharged from hospital — a follow-up study.' *British Journal of Psychiatry*, 145, pp 586–590.

JONES, K. (1988) *Experience in Mental Health: Community Care and Social policy*. London: Sage.

JONES, K., ROBINSON, M. and GOLIGHTLY, M. (1986) 'Long-term psychiatric patients in the community.' *British Journal of Psychiatry*, 149, pp 537–540.

KATSCHNIG, H. and KONIECZNA, T. (1989) 'What works with relatives?' *British Journal of Psychiatry*, 155 (Supplement 5), pp 144–150.

KEISLER, C. A. (1982) 'Mental hospitals and alternative care: non-institutionalization as potential public policy for mental patients.' *American Psychologist*, 37, pp 349–360.

KORER, J. and FITZSIMMONS, J. S. (1985) 'The effect of Huntington's Chorea on family life.' *British Journal of Social Work*, 15, pp 581–597.

KREISMAN, D. and JOY, V. (1974) 'Family response to the mental illness of a relative: a review of the literature.' *Schizophrenia Bulletin*, 10 (7a, 11), pp 34–57.

KREITMAN, N. (1964) 'The patient's spouse.' *British Journal of Psychiatry*, 110, pp 159–173.

KUIPERS, L. (1979) 'Expressed emotion: a review.' *British Journal of Social and Clinical Psychology*, 18, pp 237–243.

KUIPERS, L. (1987) 'Depression and the family.' In J. Orford (ed), *Coping with Disorder in the Family*. London: Croom Helm.

LAING, R. D. and ESTERSON, A. (1964/1982) *Sanity, Madness and the Family*. Harmondsworth: Penguin.

LEFF, J., BERKOWITZ, R., SHAVIT, N., STRACHAN, A., GLASS, I. and VAUGHN, C. (1989) 'A trial of family therapy v. a relative's group for schizophrenia.' *British Journal of Psychiatry*, 154, pp 58–66.

LEFLEY, H. P. (1987) 'An adaption framework: its meaning for research and practice.' In A. B. Hatfield and H. P. Lefley (eds), *Families of the Mentally Ill: Coping and Adaptation*. London: Cassell Educational Ltd.

LEHMAN, A. F., WARD, N. C., and LINN, L. S. (1982) 'Chronic mental patients: the quality of life issue.' *American Journal of Psychiatry*, 139 (10), pp 1271–1276.

LEVIN, E., SINCLAIR, I. and GORBACH, P. (1983) *The Supporters of Confused Elderly People at Home: Extract from the main report.* London: National Institute for Social Work Research Unit.

MacCARTHY, B., KUIPERS, L., HURRY, J., HARPER, R. and LeSAGE, A. (1989a) 'Counselling the relatives of the long-term adult mentally ill: I. Evaluation of the impact on relatives and patients.' *British Journal of Psychiatry*, 154 (June), pp 768–775.

MacCARTHY, B., LeSAGE, A., BREWIN, C. R., BRUGHA, T. S., MANGEN, S. and WING, J. K. (1989,b) 'Needs for care among the relatives of long-term users of day care. *Psychological Medicine*, 19, pp 725–736.

McCREADIE, R. G. (1982) 'The Nithsdale schizophrenia survey: I. Psychiatric and social handicaps.' *British Journal of Psychiatry*, 140, pp 582–586.

McCREADIE, R. G., WILES, D. H., MOORE, J. W., GRANT, S. M. et al. (1987) 'The Scottish first episode schizophrenia study: IV. Psychiatric and social impact on relatives.' *British Journal of Psychiatry*, 150, pp 340–344.

MANDLEBROTE, B. and FOLKARD, S. (1961) 'Some factors related to outcome and social adjustment in schizophrenia.' *Acta Psychiatrica Scandinavica*, 37, pp 223–235.

MECHANIC, D. (1986) 'The challenge of chronic mental illness: a retrospective and prospective view.' *Hospital and Community Psychiatry*, 37 (9), pp 891–896.

MILLER, D. (1987) *Living with AIDS and HIV*. Basingstoke: MacMillan.

MULVEY, E. P., GELLER, J. L. and ROTH, L. H. (1987) 'The promise and peril of involuntary outpatient commitment.' *American Psychologist*, 42 (6), pp 571–584.

NAMYSLOWSKA, I. (1986) 'Social and emotional adaptation of the families of schizophrenic patients.' *Family Systems Medicine*, 4 (4, Winter) pp 398–407.

NOH, S. (1985) 'Living with psychiatric patients: the relationship between family burden and mental health among family members'. Ph.D dissertation presented at the University of Western Ontario.

NORTHOUSE, L. (1980) 'Who supports the support system?' *Journal of Psychiatric Nursing and Mental Health Services*, 18, pp 11–15.

ORFORD, J. (1987) 'Integration: A general account of families coping with disorders.' In J. Orford (ed), *Coping with Disorder in the Family*. London: Croom Helm.

PARKER, G. (1985; 1990, 2nd edition) *With Due Care and Attention: a Review of Research on Informal Care*. London: Family Policy Studies Centre.

PARKER, G. (1989) *A study of non-elderly spouse carers: final report*. York: Social Policy Research Unit, University of York.

PEARSON, M. (1983) 'The politics of ethnic minority health studies.' *Radical Community Medicine*, 16, pp 34–44.

PERRING, C. A. (forthcoming) 'How do discharged psychiatric patients fare in the community?' In J. Hutton, S. Hutton, T. Pinch and A. Shiell (eds), *From Dependency to Enterprise: the challenge to policy*. London: Routledge.

PERRING, C. A., HUNT, B., PARRY, I. and O'CONNOR, T. (1987) 'A two-year follow-up study of discharged psychiatric patients'. Unpublished ms: Health Studies Unit, University of Sussex.

PLATT, S. (1985) 'Measuring the burden of psychiatric illness on the family: an evaluation of some rating scales.' *Psychological Medicine*, (15), 2, pp 383–393.

PLATT, S. and HIRCSH, S. (1981) 'The effects of brief hostitalization upon the psychiatric patient's household.' *Acta Psychiatrica Scandinavica*, 64, pp 199–216.

ROGLER, L. and HOLLINGSHEAD, A. (1965) *Trapped: Families and Schizophrenia*. New York, Wiley.

SEYMOUR, R. J. and DAWSON, N. J. (1986) 'The schizophrenic at home.' *Journal of Psychosocial Nursing and Mental Health Services*, 24 (1), pp 28–30.

SOMMER, R. and OSMOND, N. (1984) 'The schizophrenic no-society revisited.' *Psychiatry*, 47 (2), pp 181–191.

SOMMERS, I. (1988) 'The influence of environmental factors on the community adjustment of the mentally ill.' *Journal of Nervous and Mental Disease*, 176 (4), pp 221–226.

STEVENS, B. C. (1972) 'Dependence of schizophrenic patients on elderly relatives.' *Psychological Medicine*, 2, pp 17–32.

TALBOTT, V. A. (1984) *The Chronic Mental Patient: Five Years Later*. New York: Grune and Stratton.

TARRIER, N., BARROWCLOUGH, C., VAUGHN, C., BAMRAH, J. S., PORCEDDU, K., WATTS, S. and FREEMAN, H. (1989) 'Community management of schizophrenia: a two year follow-up of a behavioral intervention with families.' *British Journal of Psychiatry*, 154, pp 625–628.

TEST, M. A. and STEIN, L. I. (1980) 'Alternative to mental hospital treatment: III, Social cost.' *Archives of General Psychiatry*, 37, pp 409–412.

THOMPSON, E. H. and DOLL, W. (1982) 'The burden of families coping with the mentally ill: an invisible crisis.' *Family Relations: Journal of Applied Family and Child Studies*, 35 (3), pp 379–388.

TITTERTON, M. (1989) 'The Management of Personal Welfare'. Unpublished MS: Department of Social Administration and Social Work, University of Glasgow.

TOMLINSON, D. (1988) 'Let the Mental Hospitals close...' *Policy and Politics*, 16 (3), pp 179–195.

TWIGG, J. (1989) 'Models of carers: how do social care agencies conceptualise their relationship with informal carers?' *Journal of Social Policy*, 18 (1), pp 53–66.

TWIGG, J., ATKIN, K., and PERRING, C. (1990) *Carers and Services: A Review of Research*. London: HMSO.

UNGERSON, C. (1987) *Policy is Personal: Sex, Gender and Informal Care*. London: Tavistock.

VAUGHN, C. E. and LEFF, J. P. (1976) 'The influence of family and social factors on the course of psychiatric illness, a comparison of schizophrenic and depressed neurotic patients.' *British Journal of Psychiatry*, 129, pp 125–137.

VAUGHN, C. E. and LEFF, J. P. (1981) 'Patterns of emotional response in relatives of schizophrenic patients.' *Schizophrenia Bulletin*, 7 (1), pp 43–44.

WALKER, K. N., MacBRIDE, A. and VACHON, M. L. S. (1977) 'Social support network and the crisis of bereavement.' *Social Science and Medicine*, 11, pp 35–41.

WING, J. (1975) *Schizophrenia from Within* . Surbiton: National Schizophrenia Fellowship.

WING, J. K. (ed) (1982) *Long-term Community Care Experience in a London Borough*. Psychological Medicine Monograph Supplement 2.

YARROW, M., SCHWARTZ, C. G., MURTHY, H. S. and DEASY, L. C. (1955) 'The psychological meaning of mental illness in the family.' *Journal of Social Issues*, 11, pp 12–24.

Index

Printed in the United Kingdom for HMSO.
Dd.295189, 2/92, C3, 3390/3, 5673, 184113.